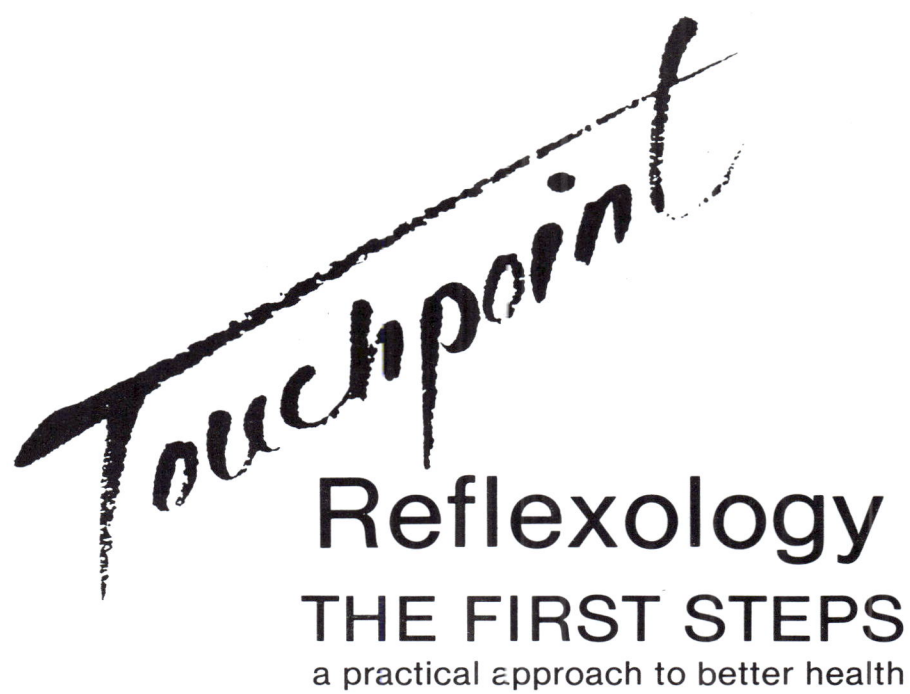

Reflexology
THE FIRST STEPS
a practical approach to better health

by Yvette Eastman

Art and Illustrations by Rosemary Phillips
Photography by Ewald Jensen

"The UN-conventional way to health"

PTARMIGAN PRESS

Dedication

Dedicated with love to
CHRIS and SAM

without whose support, love, witty comments, inspiration and patient acceptance of cold dinners I'd never have started Reflexology, never practiced it, never taught it and never written this book;

to the many folk that have sat in my recliner to share laughter and love;

to my myriad of students, so many of whom are now practitioners with their very own love seats;

to the many who made this book possible by lending me their skills in typing, illustrating, feedback, information and caring;

and to my mother who stood by me and cheered me on.

First Printing, June 1985
Second Printing, October 1987

Canadian Cataloguing in Publication Data

Eastman, Yvette, 1938-
    Touchpoint reflexology, the first steps

Bibliography: p.
Includes index.
ISBN 0-919537-23-5

1. Reflexotherapy. I. Title.
RM723.R43E28 1985   615.8'22   C85-091288-1

Ptarmigan Press
1372 Island Highway
Campbell River, B.C. Canada V9W 2E1 Canada
(604) 286-0878

Table of Contents

List of Illustrations

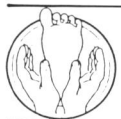

AUTHOR'S PREFACE

Success story
I have always been involved with health. As a child I nurtured animals and studied to become a veterinarian. Midway, I changed my mind to become a psychologist and group therapist. Again I changed careers to become a daycare supervisor. Then I came to a crossroad as I learned Reflexology and health maintenance. When I first came to Reflexology it was because my young son was nearly deaf. He had an eighty-five percent hearing loss, a history of painful ear infections, a voice that was painful to listen to, and, because of his deafness, mood swings when he thought others were laughing at him. Surgery was suggested, but, when I talked to others who had undergone this operation there was no great change in them. I found a Reflexologist who later became my teacher. Mrs. Kennedy worked on Chris's feet twice per week for three weeks and – he could hear! I swiftly learned this skill. My son now has perfect hearing, perfect pitch. He's a superior student with an acting career on the side. My daughter's back pain is relieved as is a bladder problem that I'd had, and, Reflexology has worked for thousands of people that I've had sessions with or those who have learned the Touchpoint method.

Touchpoint has become the most significant step in my life. As founder of the Touchpoint Canadian Institute of Reflexology, I expanded my skills to learn Touch for Health, a branch of Applied Kinesiology. I added nutritional and herbal knowledge, took Neuro-Linguistic Programming seminars, and Belief Restructuring seminars. Then, with a mix-and-match system, I blended all of the ingredients of my life to form Touchpoint. I present a portion of Touchpoint to you.

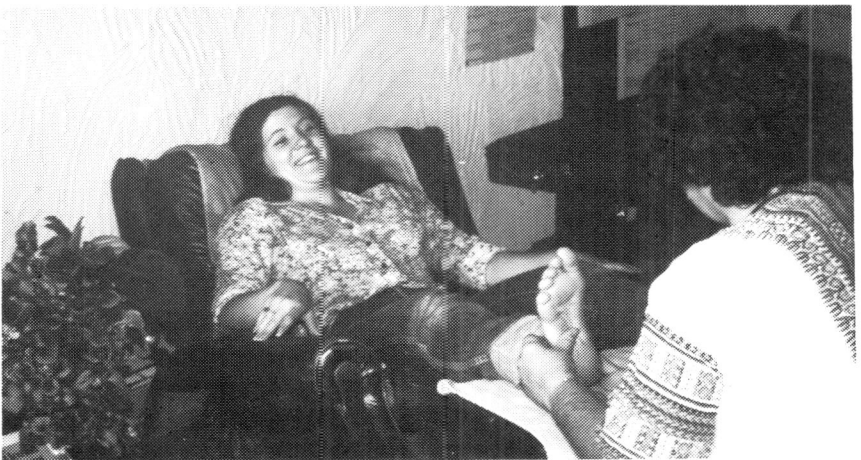

Through Touchpoint Reflexology we come to understand the complex yet simple language of the body, it's function and it's use of energy. We learn to channel that energy via reflex points. Integrating information about the organs, foods that feed them and energy expended, then the application of that information is our concern as Reflexologists, along with the alleviation of stress through a compression technique. We study the body from different angles and, once we are trained in this method, we add new methods to our knowledge to learn more about the houses we live in – our bodies. The hidden becomes obvious, the relief of discomfort becomes simple.

Experiencing is the key

Yet, with all our knowledge, experience is the key to good Reflexology. Nowhere can you be taught the fine skill of sensitivity to a reflex, nor the touch that leaves a person smiling, nor the finely tuned ear that listens not just to the body but to the person's inner voice. Hear and you will have a new friend. Remember – listening does not mean that you own the problem or that you have a need to solve it. A person needs to be *heard*. People will solve their own problems, especially if they can hear themselves speak, or receive permission to explore their feelings. Helping does not mean giving advice. No one can give the reponsibility of their physical, emotional, mental equilibrium and health to another, but as a Reflexologist you can help individuals to reach their own potential, their own strength and their own healing.

Balance is the result

Nothing can fill you with as great a sense of achievement as when you look at your friend or client whose feet have just been "well done" and you notice clear eyes, open smile, relaxed balanced features, modulated voice tones, easy laughter – and on top of it all – no pain! This is the result you wish to achieve as a Reflexologist. This is your great reward – health in all its aspects.

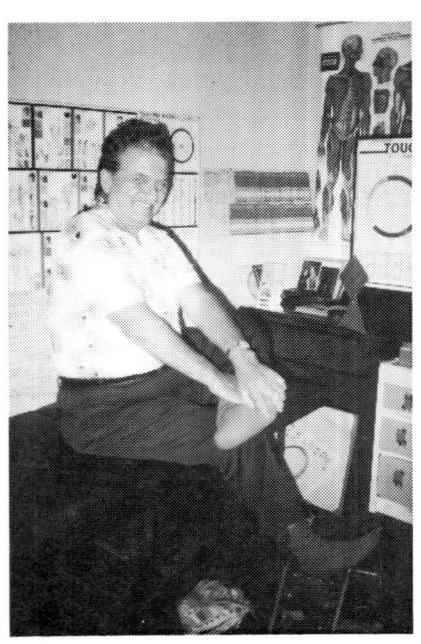

*NOTE: In writing this book, I occasionally wrote '(s)he' and sometimes wrote 'he' and sometimes wrote 'she'. My 'he' is generic – as the word 'deer' includes the word 'doe' and is a product of our language structure. '(S)he' and 'her/his' are an awkward construction so please bear with me in my use of 'he' or 'she' which I've tried to use alternately to make all of you important and to eliminate discrimination. Reflexologists come in more than one sex as do our clients, friends and the many animals who enjoy reflexology.

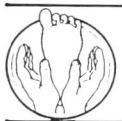

INTRODUCTION

The Placebo effect

The fact is, Reflexology works. How and why it works is now being intensively studied and interpreted. Researchers have observed and recorded the physical, mental and emotional changes that occur when Reflexology is used, but the effect that Reflexology and the Reflexologist have on these changes is still uncertain. Is it the "button" pressed that causes a response? Is it our intent, knowing what the reflex is? Is it both? Or is the answer entirely different? It may have to do with the "placebo effect" – you want to help your friend, your friend wants to please you and meet your expectations and will therefore feel better.

There are many miracle stories in diverse forms of therapy. These often occur during a public demonstration. The cripple will walk, the blind will see, the cancer victim will shed his cancer. The single mind of an audience has a keen energy that can effect a great or spectacular result. Placebo effects and miracles depend on our individual concept of what took place. Our beliefs and expectations bring about healing, forming an understanding of how healing has occured. We approach healing through our belief systems and seek aid according to that system.

Rituals and re-integration

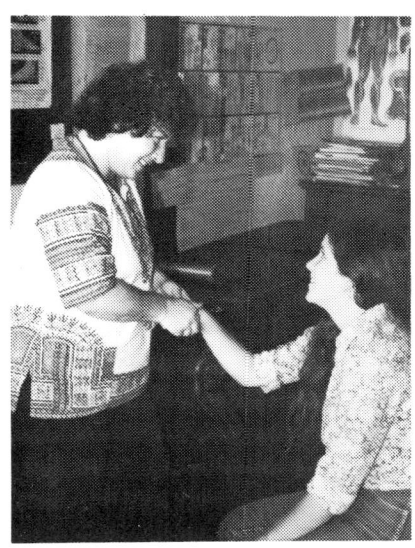

At a hospital you have a series of rituals: waiting for a bed, signing forms, cost and insurance discussion, room assignation, nurse attention, pills for sleep, pain and repair, prepping for operation, blood tests, and, notoriously poor meals. These rituals work well for those who believe in them and for ailments that can only be treated through that belief system (ie: broken bones, punctured spleen or lung).

To be an effective health practitioner of any system, you must learn the rituals which have value for both you and those who seek your aid. Each individual may require a different approach. Some approaches may seem strange because they do not yet fit with your view of the world but they do work for those who accept them. Ritual often allows people to re-integrate, to get in touch with their bodies, minds and emotions.

The Reflexology methodology, or compression technique, does the same. Sometimes a person feels better for just walking into your office. Another will require more and yet more because the touch alone was intrinsic to his awareness. Only when you touched him did he feel himself and when you were finished he may have felt desolate and disconnected.

Trust is a major key to health. Trust in self is the ultimate aim. We are stepping stones in that process. People place themselves in our hands, literally. Fear and loss of trust inhibit the the giving and receiving of healing. Exchange of trust, friendship and information will aid that trust, destroy fear and re-create health.

Re-connection and health

Our job is re-connection, the ability to put people in charge of all the events in their lives – health, wealth, success, joy, and, especially, their own recuperation. For their health we can teach them which point to continue working to accelerate their progress, reduce discomfort, remove despondency and regain their self-trust, self-health and self-love.

Work on the feet. That is your skill now. Does your friend need more? Use music, or silence, or conversation. Does your friend need even more? Work on the hands, the shoulders, the back, face, ears and more. Expand your knowledge and health sense into new dimensions with new techniques.

You can't help everyone

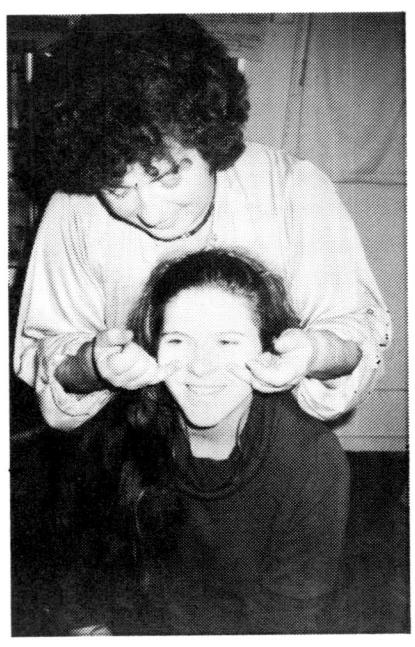

There will always be those who you can't help personally. Perhaps your ritual does not fulfill them but they can get well with another belief system. Be prepared to send them to another, whose system might be more effective for them. Learn the healing network in your community. With many integrated minds all directing positive energy for the individual it will benefit the whole of society, causing great changes on a universal scale.

Share what you abound in and it will be yours. You have all that you need to be complete. Learn to remember what you already own and let go of all the things that come between you and the surrounding universe. Allow as much ritual as the individual needs. This will prod her own healing function and affirmation of life.

Wellness is wellness, from any source. And from this source, as teacher and practitioner of wellness services, I extend my love and trust in you and your abundance on every level. Eventually, ritual will be shed and we will all be healthy because it is *NATURAL* to be *HEALTHY* in a *HEALTHY UNIVERSE*.

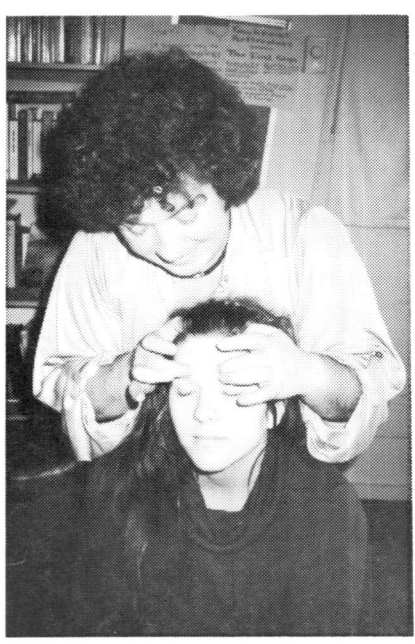

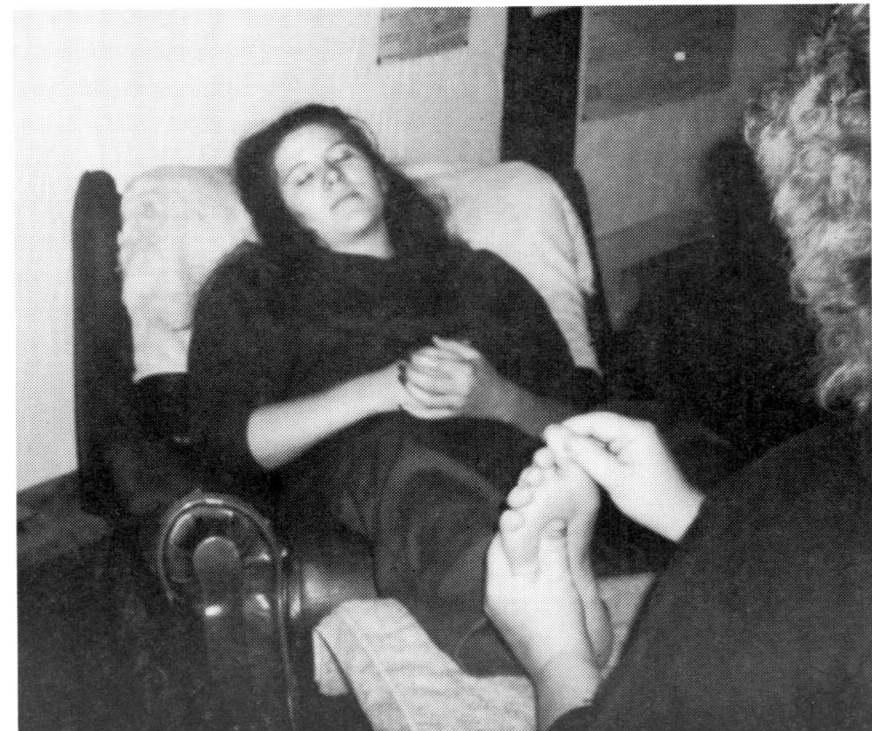

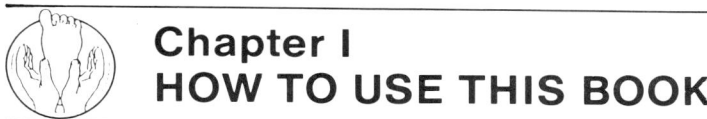

Chapter I
HOW TO USE THIS BOOK

This workbook, either alone or together with the Touchpoint Basic and/or the Advanced Reflexology Seminars or the video presentation "The First Steps" is designed to give you a complete Reflexology course.

It has been prepared with both the novice and the experienced practitioner in mind to give you a greater understanding of the reflexes in the foot and hand, their correlation to the body, how sets of reflexes work together, with specific information on how to compress each reflex. The purpose of the entire package is to put you back in charge of that "simple complexity" – your body.

To get the most benefit out of this Touchpoint workbook, a few hints are presented:

Find the Reflex

Get a "feel" for the Reflex

1. As you read about each reflex, note where it is on your own foot and on your friend's foot. Get the *feel* of *hooking* a reflex *dead on*. Then move off the reflex by ⅛ of an inch – get the *feel* of the wrong place. Now go back to the right place. Check the feeling again. Does it *feel right*? Then you've got it.

Know the parts of the book

2. Become comfortable with the divisions of the book so that you can refer to the part that serves your particular needs at that specific time.

Answer the questions

3. Interspersed within each chapter are question pages. For the most efficient personal results answer them, using both you memory and a search of the preceding pages. It's OK to get the answer wrong – that's how you learn. If you know something you don't have to learn it. If you don't know it and recognize that you don't, re-reading the necessary passage will set it in your mind. (You didn't *know* how to ride a bicycle before you rode it, you learned from the mistakes, the bumps, scrapes and falls – but WOW when you finally knew it, how free you became!) It's not always necessary to know everything by heart, if you know where to find it.

Colour the diagrams

4. Colour the pages, even the upside-down ones. One reason to colour them in, from that point of view, has to do with the left-brain function and brain integration. Colour in with a colour code for different systems. Colouring anchors the reflex in your mind and when the entire picture is colour-coded, you can easily differentiate reflexes and systems.

Record sensitive reflexes

5. Copy the back page to mark sensitive reflexes that you find on yourself or on others until such time as you can recall them easily, or to keep a record of progress. Within a certain time you'll notice correlations between the weak reflexes and certain body sensations that the person has.

Use the "note" pages

6. Fill in the blank *note* pages with your own discoveries, your own ideas and *extras*. Reflexology need not be static. As you learn and discover, new ideas will be born along with new reflexes and new methods. Keep track of them. Add in ideas from other methodologies, mix-and-match, and come up with a *newborn* idea. Then, write it up and send it to Touchpoint for publication. Bring it before us at the Touchpoint Annual Meeting to get new ideas tried out and experimented on by others. Thus, Reflexology grows. Remember – growth is change! A methodology that does not allow movement or input from other theories is on the way to slow death.

Step-by-step guide

7. Play with the "Step by Step" portion of the book. It is *just* a guide – *not* a formula. My preferred session allows my hands to go where they are most needed, and somehow they have learned to also go down the foot, working each reflex, forgetting none. Remember to *always "do"* the entire foot, returning to reflexes that need a bit more. My strategy is to alternate from plantar surface to dorsal surface in order to alternate the use of thumbs and index fingers, and to relax one hand totally while the other is busy, so as not to tire either. At first, follow the "Step by Step" program, then find your own most comfortable way.

Pace yourself to enjoy learning

8. Read at your own pace, either slowly and carefully, a little at a time or, swiftly scanning in twenty minutes. Each of us has a different *remembering strategy*. Find a strategy that already works for you in another field and adapt it to this one. Some people use a tape recorder that plays at night. Some watch TV as they study. Some use music in the background. But if your strategy doesn't work for you it's time to change it. *TRUST YOUR KNOWLEDGE – YOU ALREADY HAVE ALL THE ANSWERS YOU SEEK! ABOVE ALL – HAVE FUN!* Remember: your memory is always 100%. It's your recall that sometimes fluffs! Repetition is the key to recall and repetition is the mother of skill.

All this adds up to a fun way to use this book – fun use of Reflexology and delight as you bring all your knowledge to the forebrain then direct it to the fingers to make a Touchpoint with another.

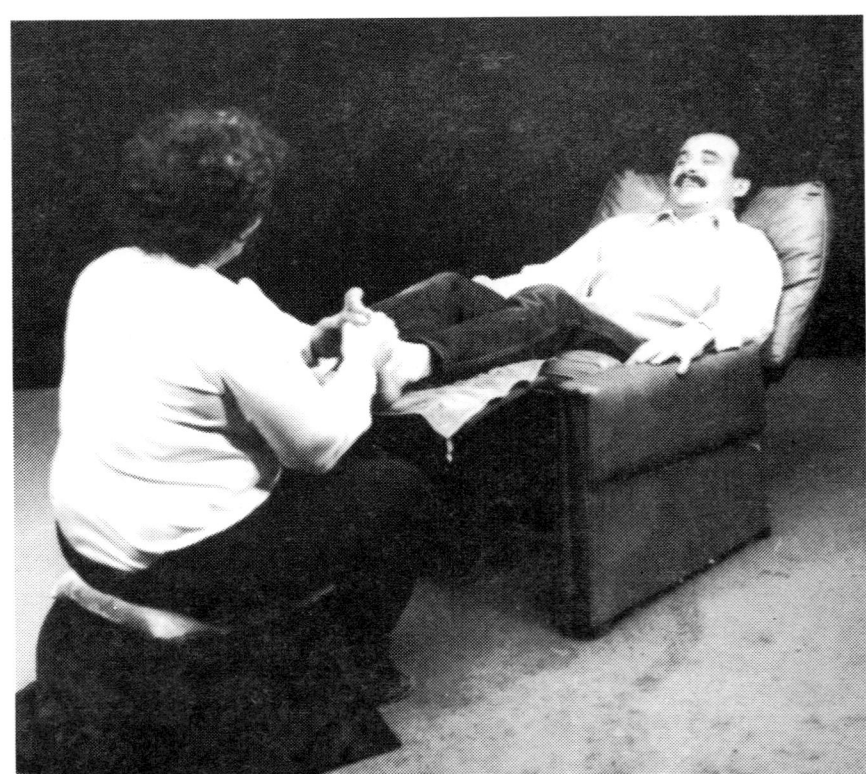

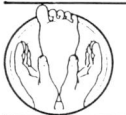

Chapter 2
WHAT IS REFLEXOLOGY?

Definitions

1. REFLEX/OLOGY
   RESPONSE/STUDY *or*

2. Reflexology is the study of the reflexes of the feet corresponding to every part of the body. Working on these reflexes relaxes tension and helps the body to seek it's own equilibrium: *or*

3. Reflexology is a compression technique used on the feet, hands or other parts of the body where there are energy points that relate to all organs and all parts of the body. When these points are contacted they unblock congestion in the corresponding region of the body so that circulation improves, elimination improves as tension is reduced, and the body normalizes and rebalances; *or*

4. Reflexology is a compression technique used on the feet that affects the whole body, reversing the effects of stress; *or*

5. Reflexology is a compression technique applied to specific points (reflexes) on hands and feet that relate to all organs and parts of the body to improve circulation and elimination, normalize body rhythms and reduce stress; *or*

6. Reflexology correlates longitudinal and horizontal zones on the feet to the same areas in the body – where the feet become a map of the system. Pressure in one zone will affect that zone in the body to which it relates. It affects the endorphine secretions of the body to relieve pain and effects relaxation of the entire system, to improve the function of all systems, all parts of the body, all rhythm patterns; *or, simply*

7. Reflexology works on spots of the feet to allow you to relax and feel better.

There are many definitions to choose from. Which one works for you? Which one is most useful to describe the new skill you are learning? People will ask, "What do you do?" You will need to answer according to your mode. Reflexology is *NOT* foot massage. Massage rubs on the skin and affects muscles. Reflexology is subcutaneous and affects spots below the skin with compression, not rubbing. Massage uses oils, lotions and/or warm baths or saunas. Reflexology works on the natural dry foot without aids. Oils make your fingers slide off the reflexes and interfere with energy flow; bathing interferes with your perception of problem areas in the foot.

Reflex Buttons

You can gain immense relief from aches and pains by applying pressure to certain reflex *buttons*. Headaches, backaches and stuffed up nose can vanish almost immediately. Arthritic hands or feet may straighten or pain may be alleviated. Hemorrhoids may cease hurting and a sore throat may heal in half the time.

Sensitivity and Tenderness

Sometimes pressure on a reflex causes sensitivity. This tenderness is an ally, an indication of congestion in the system. It tells the Reflexologist to pay attention to some impaired function denoted by the specific reflex, perhaps causing unpleasant symptoms. As the congestion breaks up, wastes are carried to the proper organs of elimination, the reflex ceases to hurt and the person feels better.

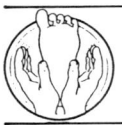

Chapter 3
HISTORY OF REFLEXOLOGY

Different Names

Reflexology has been known and used for centuries under different guises and different names from *annointing his feet with oil* to the more recent *Zone Therapy* to the *Foot lady down the road* to *Reflexology* to our own method called *Touchpoint Reflexology.*

**The old
5,000 Years Ago**

Reflexology was known 5,000 years ago in India and China, then was set aside as Acupuncture took hold. Their roots are identical. Many findings and cures are found in the Yellow Emperor's *Muangti nei Ching*, the *Book of Internal Medicine.* In acupuncture, points on meridians, or energy channels, surface on the skin.

North American Indians used pressure on the feet to relieve pain.

In Egypt, hieroglyphs and paintings have been found denoting Reflexology.

**Egyptian reflexology
treatment**
early 6th dynasty about 2,330 B.C. Wall painting in tomb of Ankhmahor, and is known as the Physician's Tomb. Translation reads:"Don't hurt me." The practitioner's reply:- "I shall act so you praise me."

Used with permission from Dwight Byers with thanks to the International Institute of Reflexology.

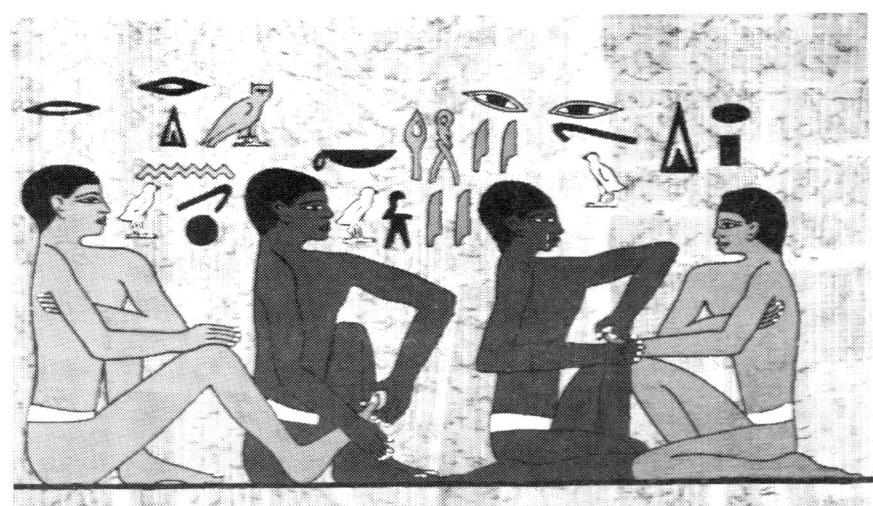

1500's   Cellini, a Florentine sculptor, used pressure on his fingers and toes to successfully relieve pain in his body.

1834   Pehi Henrik Ling, a Swede, noticed relationships with pains in organs reflected in certain areas of the skin.

1800's   An English neurologist discovered *Head Zones* and therapeutic anaesthesia was born.

1881   President J.A. Garfield of the U.S.A. applied pressure to his feet to alleviate pain following an attempted assassination.

1900's   Dr. William Fitzgerald, an ear, nose and throat specialist in Connecticut, U.S.A., replaced the use of cocaine for anaesthesia with pressure on parts of the body. He discovered the longitudinal zones in the body correlating them to the hands, the feet and the face.

1916   Dr. Edwin F. Bowers publicly described Dr. Fitzgerald's treatment, christening the science *Zone Therapy.*

1917   Dr. Fitzgerald and Dr. Bowers collaborated to write a book for doctors, dentists, gynecologists and chiropractors.

1919   Dr. Joe S. Riley was intrigued. He discovered horizontal zones on the feet and body and published a book called *Zone Therapy, Simplified*, in 1924.

1925   George Starr White added his strength and knowledge and affirmed the solidity and power of Fitzgerald's and Bower's work, pushing Zone Therapy into the limelight.

1920's   A therapist in Dr. Riley's office, Eunice Ingham, felt that, though work on the hand was effective, working on the foot, which was more sensitive, would be even better. Eunice Ingham trained in Fitzgerald's discipline, then developed her own subtle method of massage. She continued to *map* the feet, altering and developing her compression technique until it became a teachable method called *Reflexology*.

1938   Eunice Ingham published *Stories Feet Can Tell* followed by it's sequel *Stories Feet Have Told*. She taught many the skill and science of Reflexology.

Since then Reflexology has blossomed. Mildred Carter has made it a household word in the U.S.A. and Canada. Hanna Marquardt did the same in Germany. Ina Bryant talked to England. Dwight Byers, Eunice Ingham's nephew, continues her policy. Stanley Burroughs innovated with Vita Flex. Devaki Berkson added in the Yoga favour. Anna Kaye added in Polarity. Kevin and Barbara Kunz added in research and Dr. Maybelle Segal brought in simplicity.

The new   All have added, modernized and improved Reflexology, teaching it's concepts and writing books to spread the knowledge of Reflexology worldwide.

Touchpoint follows the concepts set down by all of the forerunners and in it's search to *open up* Reflexology to change, has joined to it new reflexes, new ideas, added information and new attitudes.

Touchpoint wants to *GROW* to *CHANGE*. Thanks to the efforts of its many students, the facets of Reflexology are changing as each new student adds knowledge gleaned from other professions and other methodologies to improve this one.

Our first job is to be effective Reflexologists, our second is to learn more, to innovate and create more effectiveness.

For instance, try Therapeutic Touch on the foot as if it were the model for the body – or use Applied Kinesiology, Touch For Health, or Bio-Kinesiology, in the same manner. Run meridians on the foot instead of the body. The results are amazing. Reflexology has no end – it is not stuck with a specific number of reflexes – there are more, and more. Find them! Experiment! Your practise is your testing ground – your creativeness has no limit.

And when you discover something, write us at Touchpoint, we'll publish it at our Annual Meeting, or you can present it yourself – so that Touchpoint can learn and grow – Because there is more...

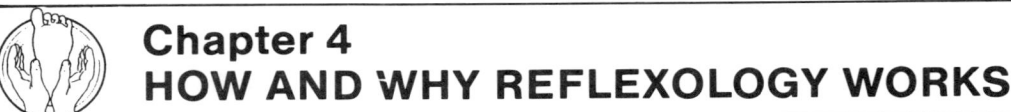

Chapter 4
HOW AND WHY REFLEXOLOGY WORKS

Energies in the body

Working on the foot rebalances the:

Chemical
Electrical
Magnetic
Thermal
and...
and...
and...

as well as energies we do not yet have names for.

All must be balanced

PSYCHOLOGICAL
emotional, mind

PHYSICAL
bones, muscles, nerves

CHEMICAL
hormones, blood, enzymes
vitamins, minerals

Have you ever

felt like this?

PSYCHOLOGICAL

PHYSICAL

CHEMICAL

Or like this?

PSYCHOLOGICAL

PHYSICAL

CHEMICAL

Fig. 1. Energy Triangle

Wouldn't it feel better to live a more balanced life, feeling good all the time?

Reflexes are below the skin

Reflexology works on subcutaneous receptors that are *below* the skin, applying a stimulus to a neuron. It works via the autonomic nervous system involving involuntary contraction and relaxation of all parts of the body.

A reflex is an involuntary response to stimulus. In Reflexology an energy current passes from a specific point in the foot, within a particular zone, to a specific organ in that zone, via a neural pathway, or an energy channel, provided there is no blockage, no congestion. An area that is blocked will affect that zone and often the zones beside it.

Afferent - efferent impulses

One possibility of how Reflexology works may be that by pressing a *reflex* on the foot you are affecting the afferent impulses (afferent – conduction inward toward a centre) travelling from nerve cell to afferent neurons which relay the message into the body and direct them to certain nerve centres or ganglia. From the ganglia, efferent neurons (efferent – away from the centre to periphery) send the impulse to an organ, muscle or gland. Messages go to a ganglia *outside* the spine. They don't go to the spine, which may explain why there is no cross-over in Reflexology – the left foot sends its impulse to the left side and the right foot sends its impulse to the right side of the body.

Longitudinal - Latitudinal zones

Another explanation may be that vertical zones carry impulses to and from the earth (energy and gravity). Horizontal zones may deal with polarity. Man is, after all, a compilation of electromagnetic energy. Tension, daily stress, causes energy blockage and stagnation which in turn can cause pain, over or under-activity of an organ, poor circulation of blood, lymph and nerves. Pain in a reflex need not point to illness – it can indicate stress. Reflexology promotes relaxation, reducing stress.

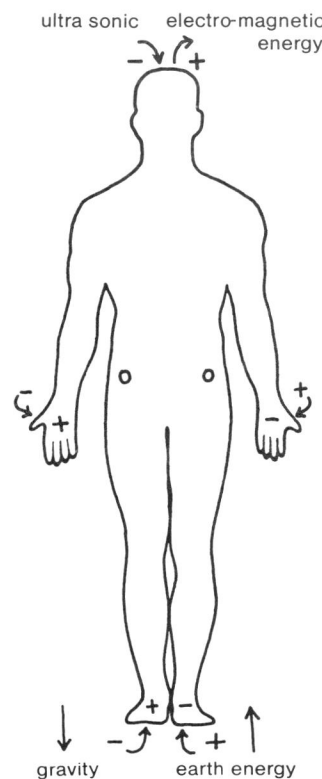

ultra sonic   electro-magnetic energy

gravity   earth energy

Fig. 2. Energy impulses.

Circulation, elimination

Or another possibility: since Reflexology promotes relaxation and circulation, if circulation feeds an organ or a cell, and it is relaxed, it will release it's waste, thereby improving elimination. When the body has proper circulation and proper elimination it is relaxed, the body rebalances and normalizes, regaining it's own individual normal rhythm.

Or, perhaps Reflexology works only on the invisible energy channels as does acupuncture. Interruption or blockage of an energy channel is like a dam in a river – causing an overflow on one side and a shallow flow on the other side of the blockage. The first stands for over-energy, the second for weakness. Compression on a reflex sends impulses that clear out the *dam* and the body resumes its flow.

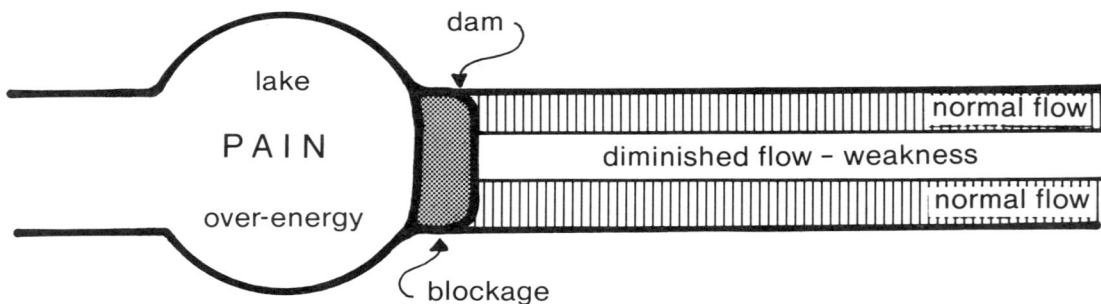

Fig. 3. Dam Model.

In the *Dam* model, if the dam is broken up, debris is pushed into the open channel, mud and gravel from the gushing lake will enter that resumed flow muddying the river and its banks before resuming its normal flow.

In the body, breaking up a blockage or congestion also leaves residue that must be dispersed and eliminated. This residue in the system may cause discomfort after a session, tiredness, nausea, headache, or *more* pain. These symptoms are temporary, especially if your client drinks more water and watches his diet until the symptoms ease. Discomfort may last two hours or may last throughout the next day.

Bio-energy

Even Westerners will admit to the correspondence of the Chinese *Yin/Yang* principles of philosophy to the sympathetic and parasympathetic nervous system and to the energy cycles within the body. Russian work by S.D. and V.Kh. Kirlian proves the reality of meridians through Kirlian photography. There is a relationship between these people's work and the term *bio-energy*, as coined by Czechoslovakian parapsychologists, a subtle form of electromagnetic waves operating in the human body.

Reflexology works

All of this is conjecture. We're left with one fact: Reflexology works. It can, in certain cases, be an analgesic (perhaps by affecting the endorphines in the system). It can repair damage to an area. It can produce health in a formerly unhealthy body. Many have experienced its benefits, as you will and as will your friends. Practice on everyone – it's a great way to make friends, though it can interfere with your dancing when you're at a party when someone mentions that you are a Reflexologist!

Occasional discomfort

The process itself may cause some discomfort as the reflexes, which are tender, are pressed, but this same sensitivity is an ally, an indication of where dis-ease is to be found. As this congestion breaks up and wastes are carried to the proper organs of elimination, the reflex ceases to hurt. It is important *not* to cause pain. It is the contact and not the pressure that brings spectacular results. Two to three pounds of pressure is more than enough. Guide yourself by your friend's comfort. Remember there is a difference between sensitivity and pain.

It is not enough to know the reflexes on the foot. The Reflexologist must learn the relationship of glands and organs affecting each other. For instance, shoulder trouble will perhaps point to gall bladder malfunction; eye trouble may tell of some tenderness in the kidney; undigested proteins in the stomach causing gas in the large intestine may cause eventual heart trouble.

As to why it works – just as in acupuncture – zones, meridians and reflex points are a mystery. Nobody knows for sure why proper pressure below the big toe affects the spinal column at shoulder level. Explanations by way of *crystal deposits* at the nerve endings of the foot that are dissolved by pressure, thereby activating circulation, are mere conjecture. They are attempts at a scientific explanation that tend to insult the scientifically trained person and antagonize him into dismissing this whole body of knowledge as trivia and wishful thinking.

The writer agrees with this point of view and leans toward a pragmatic approach: *WHAT WORKS WORKS!* If suffering is alleviated and health improved with absolutely no harm to the individual, then it should be practiced whether or not it is understood. At some future time a scientific explanation may be established. After all, limes were taken on board British ships to eliminate scurvy long before the concept of Vitamin C existed.

Tools of the trade

There are a variety of tools used in Zone Therapy. Among them are comb, rubber bands, clothespins, and rubber erasers on pencils. Often special tools are sold – wide spools, *Rollo-Flex massagers:* special sandals and foot cushions are sold in Health Food stores. This writer, as a practitioner, is totally against the usage of anything but the fingers to work a reflex, as she feels (along with most other Reflexologists) that tools might easily bruise the foot or its capillaries. The finger can pinpoint a reflex with total sensitivity to the individual being treated. I will agree to a barefoot walk on a variety of surfaces – sand, round pebbles, dirt roads, grass, and carpeting. The reflexes will be massaged naturally, sensation will be increased, musculature will improve (expecially when walking on sand). You should, however, take your shoes with you just in case the pain becomes too intense when you walk. Bruises to the foot cannot ever help a person.

As to who should receive Reflexology – *EVERYBODY* – the healthy and the ill.

After a session

After a session, the healthy will feel healthier, less tense, warmer and tingly as circulation improves. They feel lighter. If a session occurs in the morning, they feel ready to greet the world; if in the evening, they are relaxed into a restful, easy slumber. Often, old scar tissue or old bruises to one part of the body might affect another part of the body, but for the intervention of a Reflexology session. After all, good circulation is the essence of a healthful life.

Appreciate the doctor

The ill will benefit greatly from Reflexology, but keep in mind that the Reflexologist and her client work hand in hand with the doctor. The diabetic must continue to see his doctor, telling her of his treatments since they will cause large amounts of sugar to be eliminated in his urine. This will normalize. The client should not cease to take insulin until he checks with his doctor. The same holds true for the epileptic or for heart trouble or any disease where medication is taken. The Reflexologist should be aware of medication being taken so that she understands the reason for certain affected tender reflexes such as the liver or kidneys which filter drugs. Never request that a person cease to take prescribed medication. You can make her aware of the *side effects* of particular medications by showing her a book – or by suggesting that she consult her pharmacist.

Often surgery can be eliminated through the use of Reflexology, as can many diseases when organs and glands regain their normal function.

Reflexologists may work with various dis-eases from arthritis, back problems, varicose veins, digestive and eliminative disorders to heart disease, multiple sclerosis and nervous diorders and the mentally ill. For some the effect is almost miraculous. For all it is a certain benefit.

What you need to know

The Reflexologist must know far more than the reflexes of the hand and foot. She must have a working knowledge of anatomy, physiology, disease and it's ramifications as gleaned from a variety of medical handbooks. He might study related sciences such as acupuncture, acupressure, massage, and chiropractic. He can only use that for which he is certified but some of what he learns he can use, or he can refer a client to the necessary practitioner who can help in a more extensive way. For instance, where the shoulder hurts, the reflex to the gall bladder may be sensitive. After working on the foot, he may add to the session the acupressure spot to the gall bladder in the shoulder area. He may refer the client to a chiropractor where treatment to the spine might be beneficial. Reflexology sessions given before a chiropractic treatment aid the latter to *take*. In neck tension a light effleurage of the back and a holding of the muscle in spasm may relieve tension along with reflexes to the spine, solar plexus and seventh cervical.

Is Reflexology the ultimate answer?

Though the Reflexologist knows that what she does works, she does not claim it as the ultimate answer. Instead she knows that all of the sciences aid in preventive and curative medicine. She knows that doctor, surgeon, chiropractor, dentist, priest, colour therapist, physiotherapist, acupuncturist, faith healer, the client herself, and a host of others in discovered and undiscovered sciences, all contribute to the full circle of physical and mental health.

Don't prescribe, diagnose or treat for specific illness

The Reflexologist is highly involved with nutrition, with the balancing of foods, vitamins and minerals in the body. She is constantly asked for information regarding these as she works with arthritis, bursitis, colitis, intestinal disorders, headaches, migraines, and various discomforts. The Reflexologist begins to teach her clients and friends where they can find the nutrients they require, how to adapt their needs to their purses, or their tastes, what to reject, what to add. The Reflexologist is an educator of the child as well as the aged who are in hospital care. The Reflexologist learns the use of herbs as a curative and teaches it. But, as a Reflexologist, you do not prescribe, you do not diagnose, and you do not treat for specific illness.

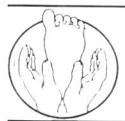

Chapter 5
POSITIONING YOURSELF AND YOUR FRIEND

Because it is important to be flexible, because we are human, three-dimensional and fluid, because "techniques" are restricting, limiting and mechanical, I am not promoting a sequential and specific method of application. When we use a particular sequence or a specific procedure, we often become stiff and angular. Fluidity is lost and dynamic interaction is obstructed.

Sit comfortably and relaxed

So instead, I will talk of positioning the Reflexologist so that she is comfortable and relaxed. Your hands "accept" the foot, cupping it, encircling it, with thumbs on the sole of the foot facing the fingers which support the top of the foot.

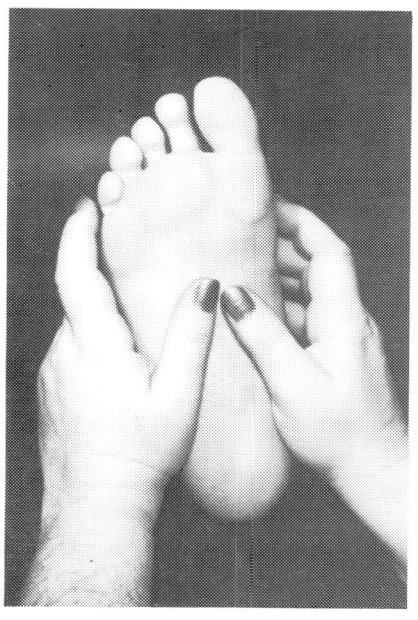

The foot is within easy reach

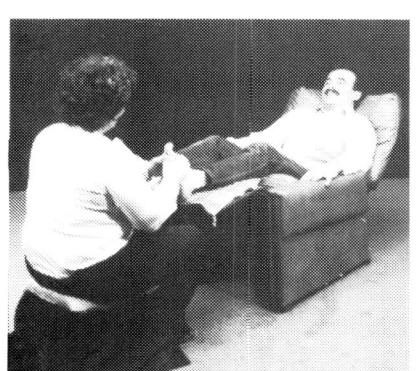

To do this, seat your friend in a recliner, on a massage table or on a surface that allows you easy, relaxed access to the feet. The foot needs to be within easy reach, neither too high nor too low, but such that your position is dictated by *your* comfort and *your* loosely flexed arms. If you are in a poor position to work, your movements become stiff, angular, uncomfortable for both of you.

You will then tire easily, your thumbs and fingers will be sore and your friend will not enjoy the session as much.

Make sure that your friend can see you. (Use pillows, if need be, to raise the head.) This will make your friend feel less vulnerable. Make sure you can see your clients face so that you are always aware of eye movements, squirms, mouth tightening, smiles that are more like grimaces – all perhaps indicating that you are working on a sensitive reflex or that you are working too hard.

Your client must be seated so that s/he is able to withdraw his/her feet, so that your friend need not feel compelled to endure pain or be at your mercy. Your client must in no way become tense, angry, alarmed, cramped, pained, anxious or frightened. All negative feelings affect the body adversely.

A clean towel under the feet is a nice touch. Since I use colour therapy as part of my work, I use coloured towels to subliminally instill the colour that I feel is needed. *(See Chapter 25, Some Effects of Colour.)*

How long?

How hard?

How often?

Building rapport

A Reflexology session usually lasts ½ hour to ¾ of an hour. Longer sessions may, in some instances, cause nausea, tiredness and other discomforts since too many toxins enter the bloodstream at once trying to be eliminated. When there is severe pain or, in the aged, the very young or in pregnancy, a session is generally shorter, compression is gentler but you may wish to work the foot more often. Adjust your session to the individual, not to the clock. Repeat the session once or twice a week when there is discomfort, less often as the person heals himself and maintenance mode when they are well. Maintenance mode differs – with some it is still weekly, with others monthly or bi-annually.

Along with his skills, the Reflexologist brings something else to the client. The Reflexologist brings ears and sensitivity. He establishes a friendly rapport that only conversation and touch can give. Conversation and caring along with Reflexology will all aid to heal the symptoms and dis-eases of a society that is under a great stress – that of a rapidly changing environment in a society unprepared to accept it's own changes. Yet we must accept the fact that tomorrow's future constantly happened yesterday. And, that too, is a cause of dis-ease.

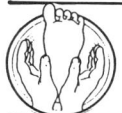

Chapter 6
USING YOUR THUMBS AND FINGERS

Remember to keep your thumb fluid and in a flowing motion. Angular thumbs may cause pain, may cause nail marks, distract the energy flow and will make your thumb sore and tired.

Both hands are always on the foot. One hand works, the other supports, maintains contact and is an expression of love, concern, and security.

All fingers may be used in Reflexology. The index will work the dorsal area, the pinky may work under the ankle bone. Use your imagination and your clients needs to decide which finger, when and where to cause the most pleasant, relaxing and health-giving experience for both of you.

Use the corner of your thumb

The corner of the thumb on the outside by the nail is the area used to *hook*, to *walk* or to *inch*. Occasionally the inner corner of the thumb is used.

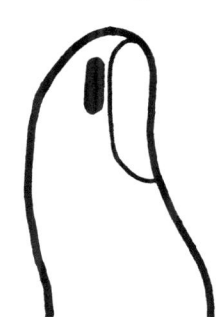

"Hooking" the Thumb

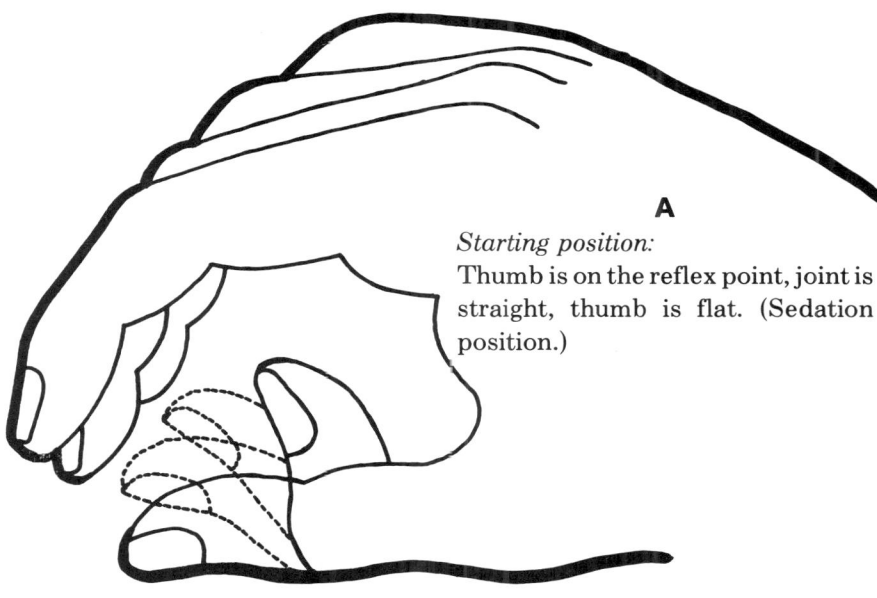

Fig. 4. Hooking the thumb.

A

Starting position:
Thumb is on the reflex point, joint is straight, thumb is flat. (Sedation position.)

B & C

Continuing position:
The thumb bends at first joint. Contact is made on the reflex point. Keep bending the thumb at first joint until it is almost perpendicular to the foot.

D

Last position:
A hooking motion with the thumb well bent at the first joint. When correctly done, as you pull back on the reflex point, the skin of the thumb will cover the nail preventing injury. (Tonifying position.)

"Walking" or "Inching"

E. *Final positions:*

The thumb straightens, maintaining contact with the reflex, then hooks again. This is a complete *hooking step*. In a *walking step*, the thumb inches in a *gathering* motion taking tiny steps forward. I call them *caterpillar steps* – little tiny inching steps, such as those used when spreading stitches to set in a sleeve when you sew – or – to movement used in *grouting* when repairing a tub. In a *hooking step* the thumb stays on the reflex, hooks in, straightens and hooks in again. The *walking step* moves forward, covering a larger area. The *hooking step* pinpoints an area that is smaller. Never *walk* backwards. Direct your walk in the direction that your nail is pointing. If you wish to change direction use the opposite finger or thumb. *Walking* the finger backwards may chafe the skin and does not hook the reflex properly.

Walk your thumb forward

NOTE: The picture shows you how to bend your thumb. It is important, however, to use the *outer* corner of the thumb by the nail. When your thumb is resting on a flat surface, *the corner of the thumb that rests on the surface is the edge that is used.* Using this corner eliminates thumb fatigue, as it is the way that the thumb normally moves towards the palm. It will also prevent *nail sticking*. Always walk in the direction that your nail is pointing.

Hook 3 times
Return 3 times

Give each reflex three *hooks*. Then go on to another reflex. Come back to each point three times. Thus the entire foot is done three times, each reflex, nine times. If a spot is sensitive, back off immediately. Keep in mind that it may hurt. Perform a relaxation exercise on the foot so the person can relax. Go to a reflex that *does not* hurt, then return to the sensitive one. *DO NOT* try to work it out all at once. Hurt takes a long time to build up and it may take a while to disappear. Use a sedation mode of compression on a sensitive reflex. Very quickly the discomfort will fade. You can use your index finger or any other finger in a similar fashion to the way the thumb is used. Starting from the straightened position, which is the passive phase, go into your hooking motion by bending the first joint of the index, middle or pinky fingers.

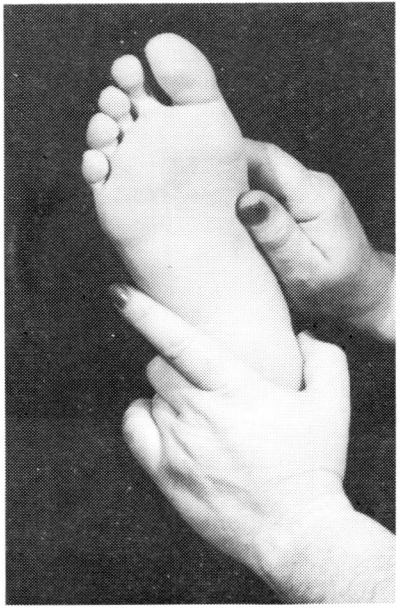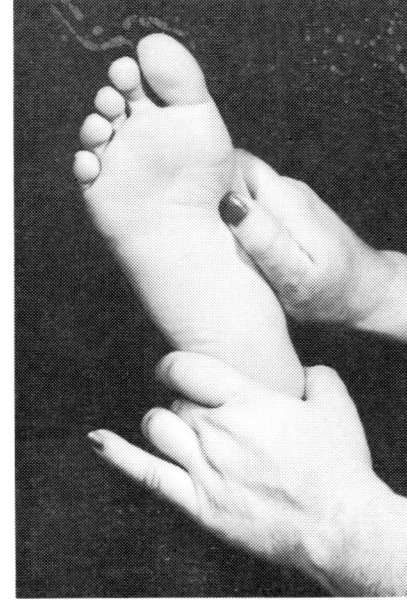

14

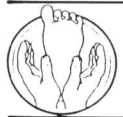

Chapter 7
THE PASSIVE AND ACTIVE PHASES

TONIFYING AND SEDATING

There are two phases in Reflexology, the Passive phase and the Active phase. The Passive phase is still, quiet, restful and sedating. The Active phase is energizing, tonifying, and may cause sensitivity.

Sedating - passive phase

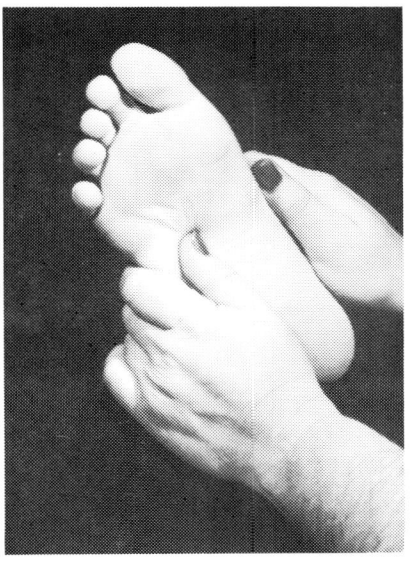

Sedating alleviates pain and calms the client, especially where there is acute pain. Use a firm hold, sustained for 2-3 minutes with an even, firm but gentle pressure on the reflex. Pain in the organ often happens simultaneously with the relief of spasm in the reflex zone. Reflexology is most effective when a second-long pressure is used frequently and interspersed with other reflexes rather than constant and in one place during a session.

On the spinal reflex, for instance, if it is painful, I often lay the entire spinal reflex of *my* thumb on my clients spiral reflex in the foot. Generally, pain subsides.

Also, when there is a painful reflex, I'll ask my client to place the tip of his tongue on his upper palate. It relieves pain and also alerts the pineal gland that healing energy is needed. But mostly, for the sedating phase, I just hold the reflex gently with my thumb or finger straight, not hooked – just hold it until sensitivity leaves.

Tonifying - active phase

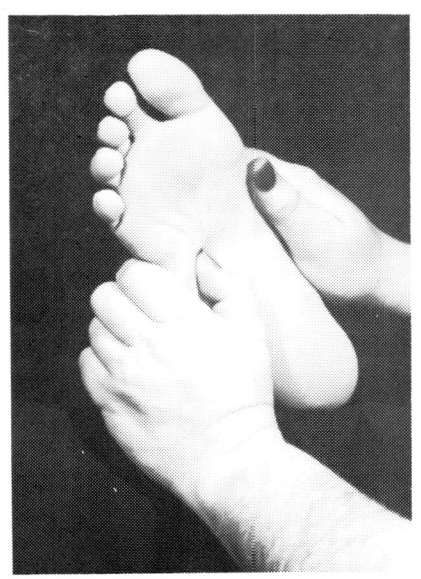

The thumb will move from a passive phase, which is relaxed and straight in position, to a curved, bowed movement (active phase) designed to enter the tissue depths, taking on strength and intensity as it continues to flex, maintaining a wide arc at its base joint. The impulse for the active phase is initiated in the palm of the hand rather than in the individual digits. If the thumb is "kinked" at right angles, the movement is incorrect, tiring, painful, and injurious. The impulse is of one-second duration and can be repeated as often as necessary.

The thumbs or fingers *always* move forward, *always* stay in contact with the surface of the skin. A client may complain of a sharp, prickling pain, thinking that the Reflexologist's nails are the cause. He is unable to distinguish pain from within his own body and pain from without. If there is pain, *BACK OFF.* Work the reflex more lightly when you return to it, if it is pressure caused. Remember, pain causes contraction of the foot and body. A tense body cannot heal. If the reflex is sore, do sedation (passive) compression instead of tonifying (active). Use delicate strength which is not bound to visible muscular power.

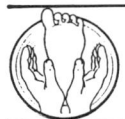

Chapter 8
ZONES OF THE BODY AND FOOT

Colour the zones of the foot and the zones of the body with different colours. Note the big toe. There are five zones in each big toe. It is in the first zone as well. Each big toe represents half of the head.

Note the overlapping in the shoulder area where zones cross into arms. How do you think that discomfort here would affect the body?

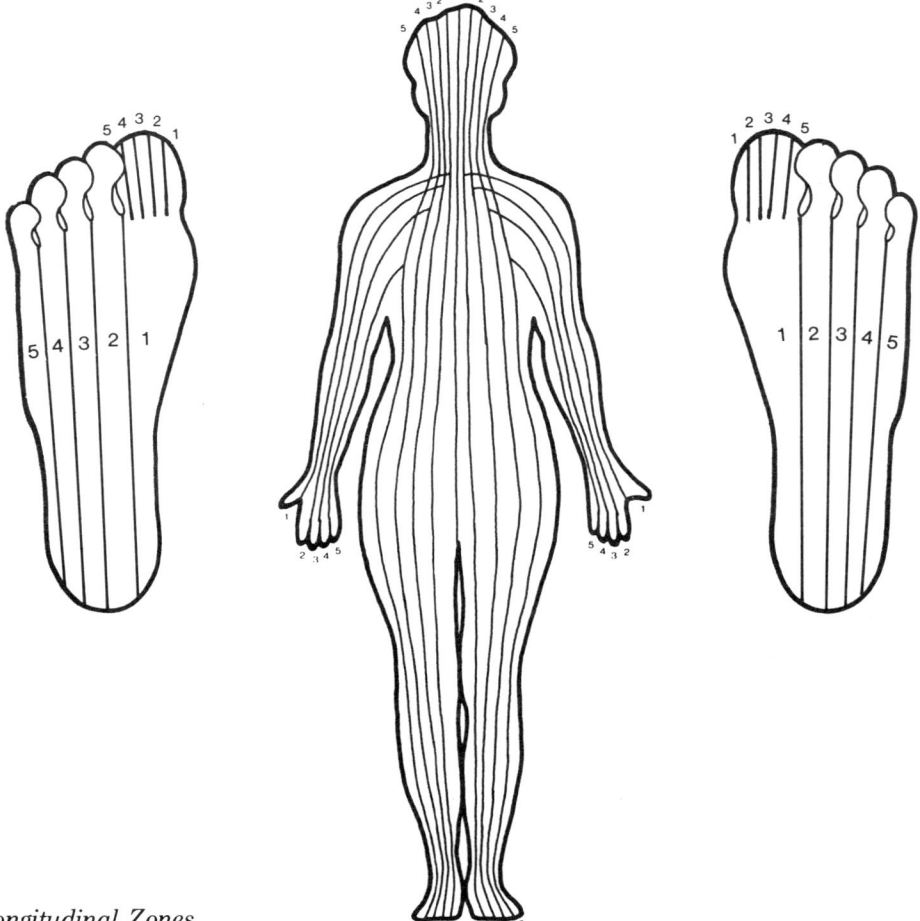

Fig. 5. Longitudinal Zones.

10 zones
10 fingers
10 toes

There are five longitudinal zones in each foot and since all zones join in the head and neck, there are five zones in each big toe and its base. They correspond to the five longitudinal zones on each side of the body. The other four toes are the *fine tuning* for the reflexes to the head and belong in zones 2, 3, 4, and 5.

The first zone is in the central portion of the head on each side of the body and goes through the centre of the neck, through both sides of the centre line of the entire body and down the inside of the thigh to the big toe. It also goes along the shoulder, down the inside of the arm to the thumb, taking in all organs or parts of the central part of the body, pineal gland, nose, spine etc.

The fifth zone starts on the outer portion of the head, goes along the outside of the body, through the outer portion of the thigh to the pinky toe. It also goes along the outside of the arm to the pinky finger, taking in the parts of the body on the outer edge of it, outer ear, part of hip, shoulder joint, etc.

Zones two, three, and four go from the portions marked in the head (2, 3, 4) to the second, third and fourth fingers and the corresponding second, third and fourth toes, taking in all organs and parts of the body that are in the 2, 3, 4 zones; kidneys, breast, stomach, intestines, etc.

This means that if you can locate an organ in the body within zones 1-5, on the left or right side, you can locate it in a zone on the foot, left or right foot. When a discomfort occurs in any portion of the anatomy, working the foot in that entire zone will bring relief.

Lateral Zones

There are six basic lateral zones: Head, Neck, Thoracic, Upper Abdominal, Lower Abdominal, Pelvic.

Arch of foot resembles spine

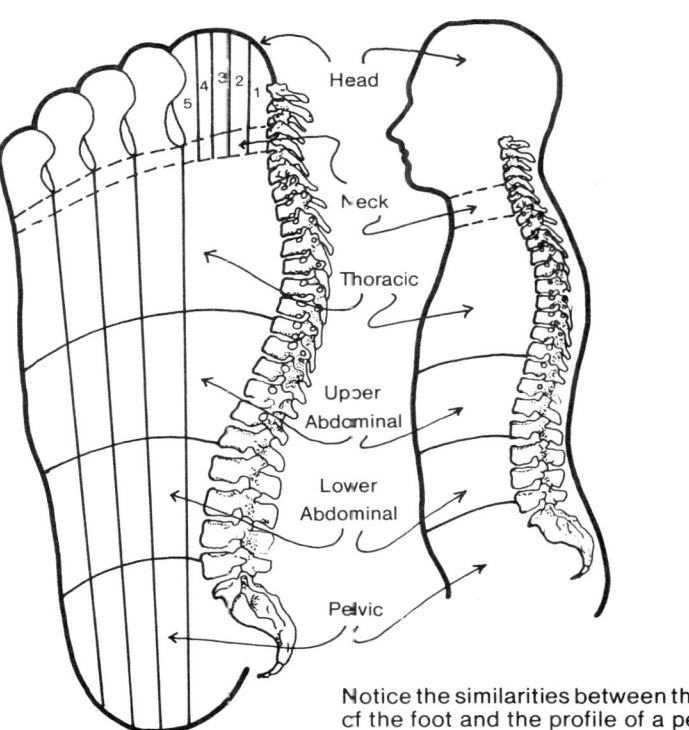

Notice the similarities between the arch of the foot and the profile of a person.

Fig. 6. Lateral Zones.

The shape of the spine corresponds to the medial side of the foot, both visually and in fact.

The toes represent the head.

The base of the toes represents the neck.

The ball of the foot portrays the chest, or thoracic region.

From the base of the ball of the foot to the waist of the foot is equal to the upper abdominal area in the body.

The waist of the foot is represented by a bony protrusion on the lateral side (pinky-toe side) of the foot, about half way down the outer edge (depending on whether the person is short or long-waisted).

From the waist of the foot to the heel depicts the lower abdomen.

The heel of the foot delineates the pelvis.

If you can locate an organ in the body, note it's longitudinal zone and it's lateral zone. You have a graph to locate the reflex on the foot within that longitudinal and lateral zone.

Other Lateral Zones

There are lateral zones that correspond to each other in the arms, legs and torso. These are depicted in *Figure 7*, below. They represent referral areas to be worked in case of injury to one portion of the body. In other words, you can work the hand for the foot, wrist for ankle, knee for elbow or waist, etc. You can also work the right side of the body for an injury to the left side and vice versa as the lateral zones reflect *across* the body.

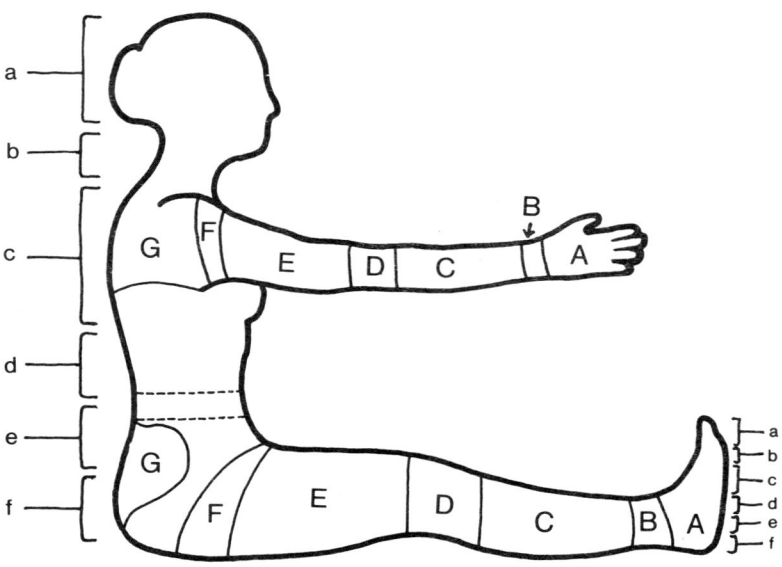

A...Hand – Foot
B...Wrist – Ankle
C...Arm – Leg
D...Elbow – Knee – Waist
E...Upper Arm – Upper Leg
F...Shoulder – Hip
G...Upper Back – Lower Back

a) Head
b) Neck
c) Thoracic
d) Upper Abdominal
e) Lower Abdominal
f) Pelvic

Fig. 7. Body Zone Correlations

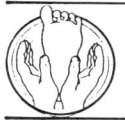

Chapter 9
A MAJOR CAUSE OF DIS-EASE – STRESS

Dis-ease demands change

All Dis-eases start with a *positive* intention.

Some part of the body/mind wants, needs, insists on *CHANGE*. Given its options, it chooses what *it* considers the best option to effect change – even though you may not consciously agree.

When the Body and the Mind disagree you have a B I N D.

Most discomforts can be traced to stress. Stress can tighten muscles, which may *squeeze* nerves, impeding the neurological impulse to organs and parts of the body, may impede blood and lymph circulation, thereby reducing flow to certain areas, and restricting elimination from others.

Stress has a particular way of affecting the system.

Stress – How It Works

Stage 1. Alert

The brain signals the body to release stress hormones into the bloodstream and to every part of the body. The blood bypasses the digestive system and floods the musculature.

The blood supply to the front of the brain (cerebral cortex) decreases, shutting down non-essential areas of the brain, stream-lining thinking processes. The sympathetic nervous system is poised for action. If stressor continues – on to Stage 2.

Stage 2. Response

Fight/flight response – choices are simple: to deal with the stressor; change if we can; avoid when we can't accept stressor; fight when we can't avoid; surrender, leave or flee when we must.

In fight response, the brain sends blood to the face, neck and chest, preparing the upper body for physical struggle. In flight response, blood is drawn away from the face, neck and chest and supplied to the arms and legs for running. In both, blood is drawn away from frontal lobes, interrupting the intellect and thinking processes, leaving the unconscious in charge. If stressor continues and we can't cope – on to Stage 3.

Stage 3. Overwhelm

We are rattled, off balance, blank, falling apart, at wits end. The body's goal is to prevent fatal overloads of stress. Disorientation is a protection. Overwhelm demobilizes. Blood is drawn back from the limbs and sent to the abdominal organs. The liver, lungs and kidney remove stress hormones. The arms and legs become hard to move; slow-down-and-rest is the result. Poor circulation to the brain reduces mental capacity, preventing reaction. Mistakes, accident prone-ness, and procrastination can result. If serious, mental fogging, dizziness, inattentiveness, fatigue, a heavy feeling in the belly (where the blood is) and fainting can result.

Chapter 10
STARTING REFLEXOLOGY

Addressing the client

Reflexology is a science that deals with the principle that there are particular spots or *reflexes* in the feet and hands that relate to each organ and each part of the body.

Energy uses these reflexes as channels to these areas to relax them, improve circulation to them, improve elimination from them and return the body to its rhythm.

Don't say to a client:

"Sure, I can fix that in no time."

"Of course I can help your arthritis, diabetes, back problem, numb fingers, cold nose."

"It will take ten treatments to cure you."

We are not doctors. We cannot treat, cure or diagnose.

Say, instead:

"I've worked with several (many, a few) people with that problem and *they* have had a lot of success!"

"Let's work on your feet and see what *they* have to say."

"I'll do your feet and *you* tell me the result."

"Most people can tell how often to get their feet done and how long to come. Your feet will probably tell you."

REMEMBER: You are a channel for stress reduction. People heal themselves, expecially if the option for health is a better one than the option they have and, if their dis-ease does not have secondary gains.

Reflexology DOES NOT:

DIAGNOSE
PRESCRIBE
TREAT A SPECIFIC ILLNESS
CURE

Reflexology DOES:

IMPROVE CIRCULATION
IMPROVE ELIMINATION
IMPROVE RELAXATION
RETURN THE BODY TO ITS
    NATURAL RHYTHM

If there is sensitivity when pressure is applied to a reflex, the related organ is congested.

When you are hurt or tense you could

squeeze it
  nibble at its edges
    rub it   nurture it
      stroke it   dilute it
        medicate it   bite it   love it
          mask it   hurt it   cool it
            cover it   concentrate on it   warm it
              ignore it
                live with it   OR...

YOU
    COULD
        USE
            REFLEXOLOGY!

Questions

1. We use a _____ technique on the reflexes to effect these changes.

2. The cause of most ills is _____.
    Stress causes congestion as well as pain, often in a distant portion of the body.
    Other causes of congestion are: _____.

3. How hard? _____

4. How often? _____

5. How long?_____

You can often guide the length of a session or work to a particular area by the amount of sweating that occurs. Often, when the foot, or part of it, is done enough it sweats.

Decide (internally) what is happening in the body to cause these relationships of sensitive reflexes.

Choose to work more on sensitive reflexes and associated reflexes.

Recognize problems that affect the foot (puffy bladder reflex, dropped arch, bunion, callouses on heel, by big toe, on the ball of the foot, hammer toes, injuries to foot).

More questions

6. How do each of the above affect the body? (To answer this question think of the benefits as well as the detriments to the person.)

Decide whether the person you are working with needs more sessions.

7. What do you answer when a reflex is sensitive and the person asks, "What was that?"
8. Answer the question, "What's wrong with me?"
9. Answer, "Should I stop my medication?"
10. Answer, "The doctor says I have X disease, what do you think?"
11. Answer, "Should I have the operation my doctor says I should have?"
12. Answer, "What should I do?"
13. Answer, "How long will it take to cure me?"
14. Answer, "Will vitamins and Reflexology fix me up?"

Answer wisely so that you state your thoughts, offer no suggestions, no directions, prescriptions, treatments and still support and help them and... keep a client.

Consider these statement/questions

"Wouldn't you be surprised if you woke up on Wednesday and you felt excellent?" (Your back felt fine etc...) If the answer is "Yes, I'd be surprised" that person will probably feel exquisite on Wednesday. Or, if you feel confident, tell your client that the session is free unless she is *not* fine by Tuesday, then she owes you X dollars. *IT WORKS!*

21

More questions

1. You can overwork the feet causing discomfort. TRUE____FALSE____
2. What is Reflexology and how does it work?
3. You should always try to work out painful reflexes. TRUE____FALSE____
4. Name three key points for relaxation. _____

    _____

5. What disease is most readily cured by Reflexology?
6. Give three reasons why the foot is important.
7. It is important to follow a step-by-step order as you work down the foot.
    TRUE____FALSE____.
8. Rituals are of little importance in the healing process. TRUE____FALSE____
9. Stress is only involved in muscular or nervous discomforts.
    TRUE____FALSE____

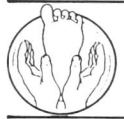

Chapter 11
DESCRIPTIVE WORDS AND EXPRESSIONS

Effleurage	firm pressure
Petrissage	kneading
Friction	large kneading
Tapotment	percussing
Stimulation	holding contact, gentle movement
Specific compression	hold 5-15 seconds when tenderness leaves or you feel energy (pulse beat)
Inching	with fingers or nail, also called walking step when done with finger. *Nail* can *inch* across top of toes.
Breath stroke	direct to part of body (guided with patient). Command organ to relax. Breathe in colour(s) that benefit your client. Both of you can do synchronized breathing.
Affirmation stroke	"This organ which I am pressing is being healed."
Nerve stroke	touches hairs not skin, balances nervous system
Cleansing stroke	as above, 2-3 inches away from body. Clears energy field.
Stretching	stretch area to fullest edge. Maintain 15-30 seconds. Stretch a little beyond edge. Release. Works on muscles of leg and foot.
Wringing stroke	wring foot in opposite directions. Limbers foot and entire body.
Plexus pull	grasp foot, thumbs on Solar Plexus. Flex foot past right angle. Pull foot gently toward you. Have patient breathe in three times, on last breath jerk foot straight back towards you. Works on Solar Plexus, subconscious, working talus and back problems.
Lymph push pull or tendon notch stimulation	thumb in lymph notch. Move feet into full flexion (right angle) applying firm pressure. Press, release five times. Works on breathing, lymphatics.
Circular petrissage	screwing stretch on toes front-back. Works on head, neck, eyes, lymph and shoulder muscles.
Lateral petrissage	screwing stretch on toes side-side. Works on head, neck, eyes, lymph and shoulder muscles.
Venous pump	begin at heel, stretch achilles tendon. Make fist and knuckle the calf from top of tendon to knee firmly. Works on lymphatic circulation and veins.
Toe release	one thumb holds on top where toe joins foot, other hand supports foot, pull toe straight out (no bending). Stimulates tendons, clears head/neck.
Toe pull tendon stimulation	hold toe same as above but press tendon up foot to ankle on each toe. Releases tension in foot.
Toe rotation	turn all toes firmly.
Toe extension release	fingers on top of toes, press in at base. Push toes gently/firmly, stretch, hold, go further, release. Releases tension in feet and toes.
Flexion release	grip hand over toes, thumb on top of toes, fingers in lung area. Quick motion. Bend toes downward. Push arch up at lung reflex. Clears bronchial and upper back area.
Bunion smack	pull big toe out (towards other foot). Smack bunion with fleshy part of thumb. For bunions, five times a day, or for neck and shoulders.

Eye ear stretch	stretch skin from little toe towards big toe. Drains eyes, ears, sinuses. Do this after eye-ear reflexes.
Toe effleurage	work down each toe to base for veinous drainage.
Leg-wring	stimulate by wringing leg up to knee. Affects a variety of points on leg.
Menstrual point	four fingers from ankle bone
Shin bone stimulation	3-4 fingers under shin bone to knee. Circulation, blood and lymph.
Tonify stimulation	first locate *stomach 36*. When your client's hand is over the lightly bent knee, the end of the middle finger lies on *stomach 36*. Place one finger on *stomach 36* while your other hand goes along the lateral (outside) of the leg and presses below the bone, along the entire side of the calf muscle. Alternate pressure on different point on the calf with pressure on *stomach 36* to stimulate the entire system.
Endocrine stimulation (especially in stress adrenals)	stimulate centre calf points (centre of gastrocnemius) back of leg.
Plantar surface	bottom surface of the foot, that surface which you walk on.
Dorsal surface	the top, upper surface of the foot.

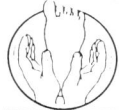

Chapter 12
DESSERTS, TREATS AND RELAXATION EXERCISES

Desserts

Desserts are gentle motions performed on the feet and legs that you can use:

1. at the beginning of a session to relax the foot, to learn about its *feel* and to allow your client to get the *feel* of you;

2. after each section of the foot is completed – big toe, toes, ball of foot, arch of foot, heel, medial side, lateral side, ankle etc...;

3. immediately, as soon as a sensitivity is encountered, to relax the person, remove the pain and regain trust;

4. at the end of a session to insure the lasting relaxation effects of Reflexology.

Observations

First check the foot for:

injuries (ask about them)

aches, pains (where, what kind, when)

scars (ask about them)

discolouration (ask about it)

are both feet different colours?

temperature on foot (is one spot cold or hot?)

are both feet different temperatures?

varicose veins, phlebitis (don't work on or near these)

operations (be aware of screws or rebuilt bones) varicose vein operations etc.

hairlessness (may indicate poor circulation)

nails (thick or shattered – poor circulation or lack of minerals, pressure from shoe)

callouses – near big toe – affects neck, near heel, affects hip or low back

plantar warts – know the name of a good podiatrist

corns – suggests irritation by footwear

First touch

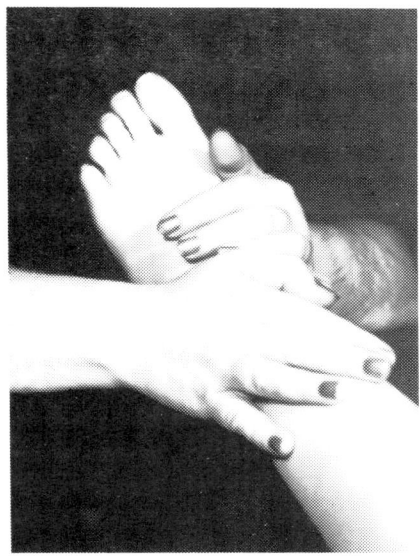

Relax the foot and let it trust you. Touch and stroke the foot sliding your hands gently but firmly up the foot with both hands, then up both sides of shin bone to the knee (effleurage). Curve down to the calf muscle and downwards to the heel and up the foot. As I go back up the foot from heel to toes, I stretch the outermost portion of the foot with my hands and almost make a snapping sound as my hands reach the top of the toes. Do this several times.

Ankle rotation

Hold your left hand so the back of it is toward you, thumb and fingers pointing down. The webbing of the left hand is over the ankle, the thumb is on the outside of the foot, fingers on the inside of the foot, thumb and index are in front of the ankle bone (toward you) and apply *NO* pressure. Pressure is across the ankle itself. Hold the big toe side with right hand and rotate the foot one way and the other or in a figure 8. Slip the left hand under the heel of the foot and rotate the *heel*, pushing *it* in a circle, streching the tendon at the back of the leg. You are looking for stress, muscle tension and edema. For the left foot, change hands.

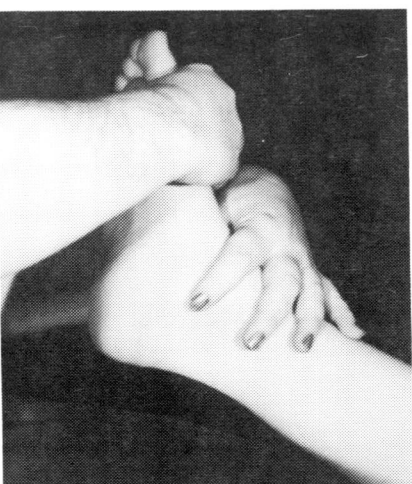 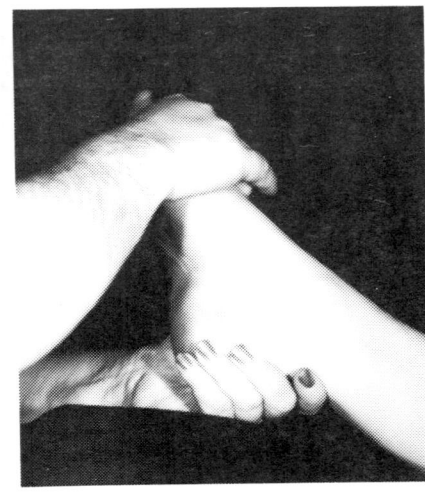

The jiggle

The hollow of the palms cradle both ankles. Pressure is applied in a back and forth motion using the heel of the thumb to push the foot to one side. Push it to the other side with the heel of the other thumb. The motion is similar to a locomotive wheel joiner. Jiggle as fast as you can. Jiggling swiftly elicits laughter, trust, allowing the person to temporarily surrender control of their feet.

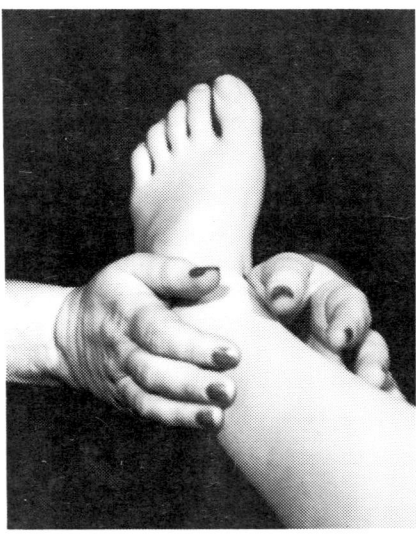 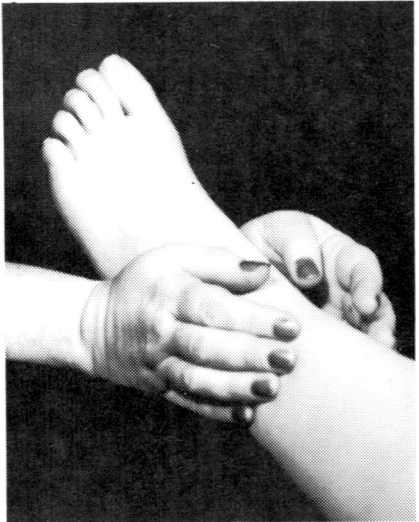

Flexion/Extention

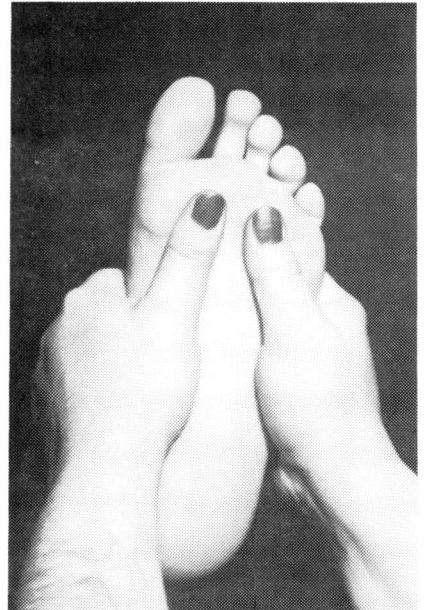

With thumbs on the ball of the foot, flex the foot to its highest point, hold it there for 8-15 seconds then push a bit more. This stretches the tendons, allowing them to relax. Extend the foot using the fingers on the top of the foot. Hold 8-15 seconds then extend more. Push the foot to one side, hold, a bit more, and the other side, hold, a bit more. All of this gives the body, leg and foot mobility and relaxation while also aiding the bladder function of the body. Do the same with the toes; this aids neck and head mobility.

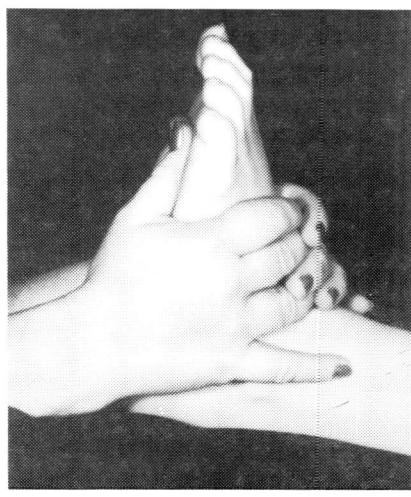 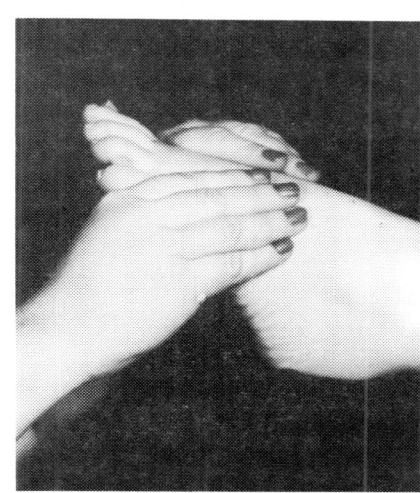

The jerk

Flex the foot again, thumbs on the ball of the foot, fingers tight against the top of the foot. Pull the whole flexed foot toward yourself gently, then give a strong, swift jerk toward yourself once. This releases the talus and the lower back.

Spinal twist

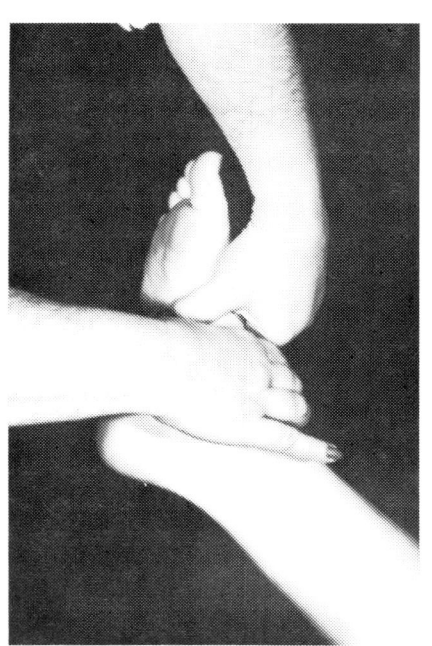

Both hands are on the medial arch of the foot, both thumbs joined in the arch on the plantar surface of the foot, with fingers on the top of the foot, hands one against the other. The hand closest to the ankle does not move, the other hand jiggles the foot back and forth, then moves toward the toes about ½ inch. The ankle hand moves up to close the gap as the toe hand again jiggles the foot, then moves up half and inch. This twist and move continues until the ankle hand reaches the bunion area below the big toe. Now the *toe* hand holds the big toe while the *ankle* hand holds the bunion area firmly. With the *toe hand*, gently pull the big toe up and turn it slowly in both directions alternately, from deep inside the bunion joint. This releases the spine and neck, relaxing it and giving mobility. Be aware of any stiffness of the big toe and relate it to the person's neck area. Twist and turn each of the toes in a screwing motion, bringing circulation to the head. Pull straight up on each toe. If they snap that's OK, but do not force them.

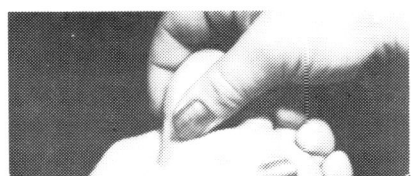 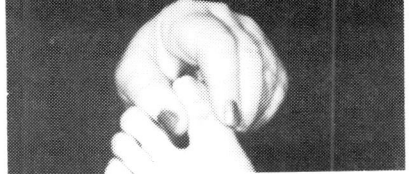

**Mind point
"Splitting" the gastrocs**

Reach up the calf to the centre of the base of the calf muscle. Find a little cave here. Hold that spot with the index or middle finger. It helps to reduce mind-induced tension. It may hurt if the person worries a lot or if she has done a lot of mental work. To *split the gastrocs* you go up the centre of the calf muscle and stretch and pull to either side of the centre, easing mind induced stress, while relaxing the calf muscle. You are using a type of kneading motion (petrissage).

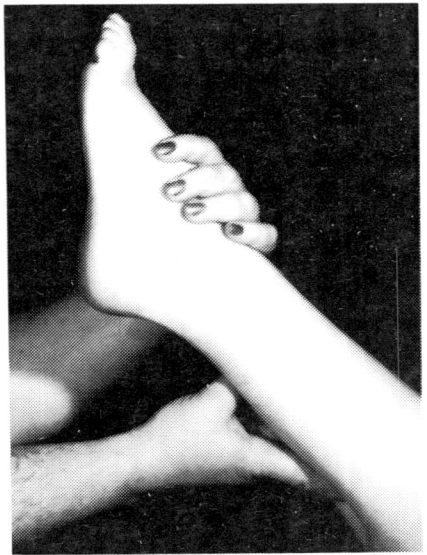

Stomach 36

Hold the *stomach 36* point, below the knee, where the person's middle finger reaches when his hand is on his knee. With the other hand, press in along the entire outside of the leg, under the bone, alternating *stomach 36* point with others. This affects the entire body, tonifying, stimulating the system.

Chest squeeze

One of the hands makes a loose fist. Place the flat upper phalanges against the ball of the foot. The other hand cups the dorsum of the foot, barely overlapping the start of the toes. Gently coordinate the hands as they push the ball of the foot away from you into the cupped hand. The cupped hand now gently squeezes the top of the foot toward the waiting fist. Both of the hands are in constant contact with the foot, and alternately push and squeeze in a kneading undulating fashion. This relaxes the chest, back and the whole upper half of the body. You can continue the *chest squeeze* motion down the entire foot.

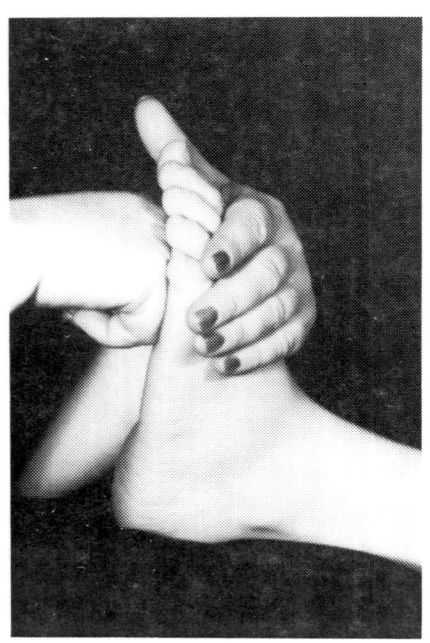

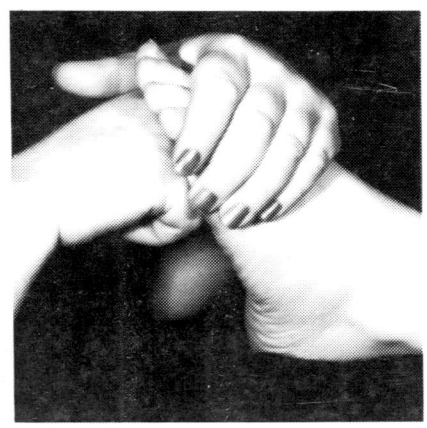

Back scratch

Use the backs of the nails along the whole top of the foot toward the heart in a gentle scratch. This calms the stomach in motion sickness, heartburn, nausea. Some people react badly to this dessert, so check with them first to see if it irritates them. The same dessert on the *hand* works for car sickness and infant colic.

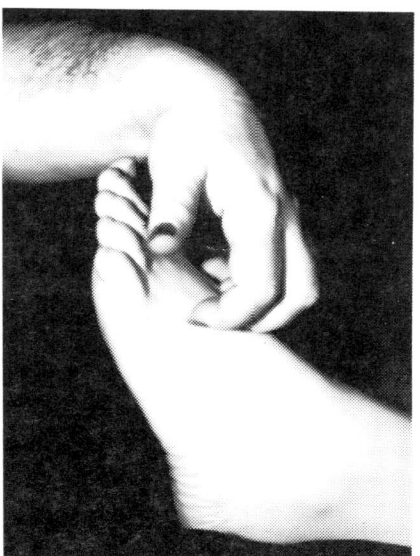

Solar plexus

Do this at the start of a session if the person is very nervous, in pain, stressful, or ticklish. Do this at the end of a session with the breathing technique and several times during a session without the breathing technique. Hold the base of the ball of the foot, right in the centre where there is a little depression. Do both feet simultaneously, one thumb on each foot. This reflex is *ALWAYS* done on both feet simultaneously. Hold gently but firmly until the person sighs or appears more relaxed.

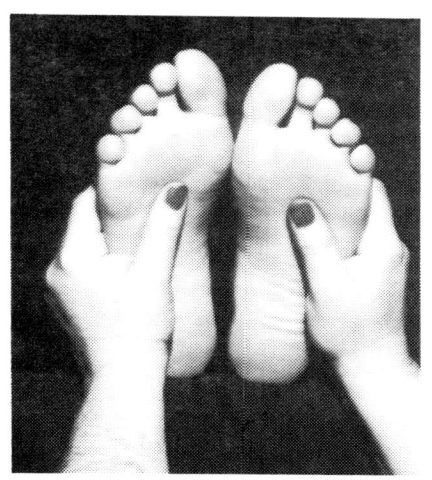

Solar plexus breathing

At the end of a session have the person breathe in deeply 3 times and ask them to hold the 4th breath as long as comfortable, then gently stroke downwards as they exhale.

The ability to hold one's breath is often affected by the stomach and pancreas function.

Often after *solar plexus breathing* the client will feel tingling in the hands and feet, lightness in the head, and may begin to perspire, especially in the extremities. The reason behind this is that working the *solar plexus* brings circulation to the extremities, dilating capillaries, and improving nerve impulses.

7th cervical/coccyx

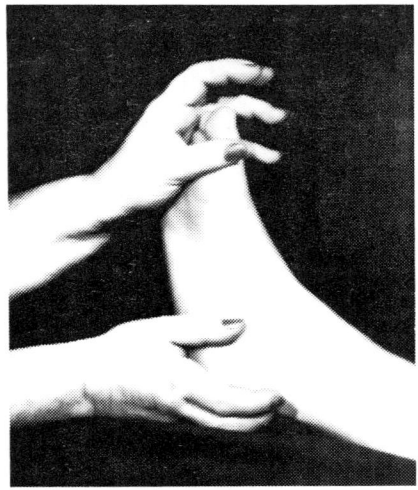

Hold the *7th cervical* reflex at the side base of the big toe and the *coccyx* reflex at the side edge of the beginning of the heel just beyond the arch of the foot. Hold both spots simultaneously, very lightly, until you feel either energy or an even, synchronized pulse in both reflexes. Use this at the end of a session to balance the flow of energy in the whole body. If the pulses are slow to synchronize ask your friend to breathe energy into his body from the feet up through the spine (or from the head down, as you wish).

Wringing stroke

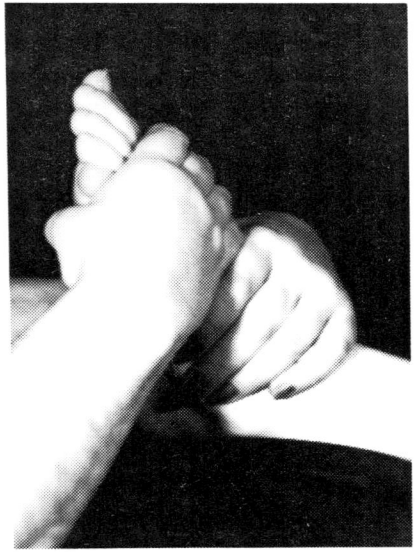

Twist the foot as if you were wringing a dishrag, with one hand wringing upwards, the other downwards, then reverse. This relaxes the foot, the spine, rendering fluidity to the body. Wring the foot upwards, thumbs on the ball of the foot, fingers on the dorsal part of the foot. This improves the persons gait.

Percussion

Tap/slap the foot gently all over. This improves circulation. Use your hands, finger tips, and a cupping movement (hand partially closed so that finger tips and heel of hand make contact).

Nerve stroke

Touch the hairs, not the skin. This brings the nervous system into balance.

Cleansing stroke

Touches from 2-3 inches *away* from the foot. This cleans and clears the energy field and is used at the end of a session.

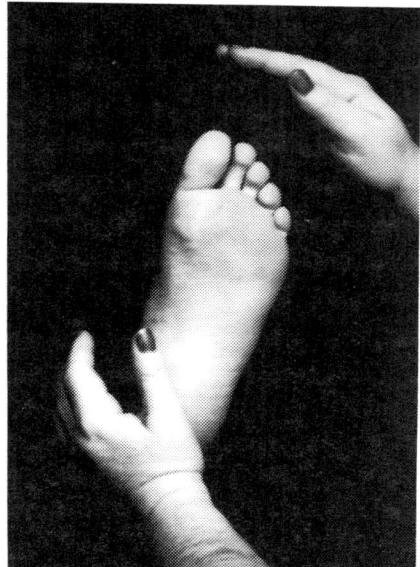

Colour breathing

Check *Chapter 25, Some Effects of Colour,* or use your own knowledge of colour. Either send colours into the system, or to particular areas – or ask the person to breathe in one colour (beneficial) and breathe out any visualized colour that is less than excellent. For example, breathe in laser blue into a painful area, breathe out the black, muddy green, red, or whatever shade your friend perceives at that pain spot. Ask the person, "If your hurt knee had a colour, what would it be?" (Answer – grey.) "And what colour is your healthy knee?" (Answer – blue.) "What would it take to change the grey to that shade of blue?" (Answer – pink and blue.) Breathe in pink and blue, breathe it into your knee and as you breath out – blow out grey. (Repeat until the colour is uniform.)

People love desserts

Now you're ready to work on the foot after having used at least five or six desserts at first to relax and prepare the foot. Repeatedly intersperse other desserts throughout the session when the person tenses or if a reflex has been sensitive. People love *desserts* so use a lot of them.

Questions on relaxation exercises and desserts

1. Why is the first touch so important?
2. It is important to perform at least 10 desserts prior to working the foot. TRUE_____FALSE_____
3. If a person has a sprained ankle work the ankle anyway, but be gentle. TRUE_____FALSE_____
4. Desserts are pleasant and relaxing but serve no other purpose. TRUE_____FALSE_____
5. Which dessert is used for ticklish people?_____For a person whose feet are very sensitive?_____
6. What is the purpose of the *7th cervical/coccyx hold?*
7. Which dessert(s) affects the lower back?
8. Which desserts bring circulation to the head?
9. Which dessert is useful in motion sickness and infant colic?

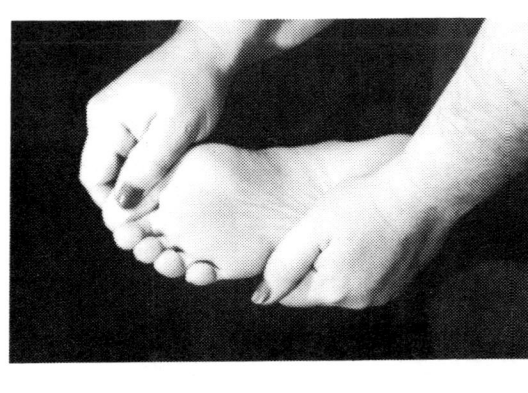

Chapter 13
ARCHITECTURE OF THE FOOT

Organs, glands and parts of the body as represented in the foot reflexes.

The following is a breakdown of the reflexes, the organs and parts of the body they reflect to, and a specific method of compression for each. It also gives some nutritional ideas. Work lightly, gently, caringly and be specific with your contact points. Remember, it is the exact contact, not the pressure, that is most effective. Pay special attention to sensitive reflexes. Come back to them often but do not use tonifying active phases continuously. Work each reflex three times and return to each three times (nine in all). Work more often and lightly on the sensitive ones. Within the description of the function of each gland and part of the body are many clues as to the associated reflexes to work. Draw conclusions, try them out on yourself and your friends.

The order presented is the one show in *Chapter 28, A Reflexology Sitting – Step by Step.* This will facilitate the locating of those reflexes.

Name of Organ -location -system	Function of Organ -supplement (food)	How to Locate and Work the Reflex
Pituitary Gland -base of the brain -both feet *endocrine system* 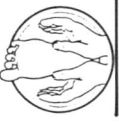	The master endocrine gland, regulates growth, hormone activity of all other endocrine glands, milk secretion, endorphine secretion, it regulates sexual activity and timing, regulates ovulation cycle, interacts with the nervous system. It affects muscular strength, dilates arteries (as in headaches) and affects fever. -Vitamin A, Manganese	Find the centre of the *whorls* on the big toe (often located near the second toe), feeling for the little cave under the skin. Thumb is straight with only the ouside corner, by the nail, touching the reflex. Bend thumb, while anchoring the fingers on the side of the big toe, then pull the cave-like reflex towards the centre of the big toe while applying pressure in the big toe.

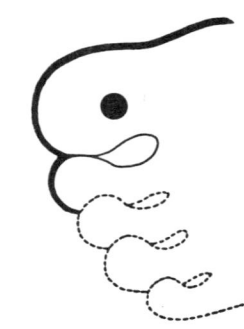

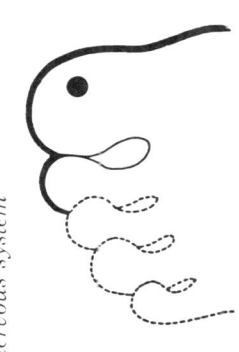

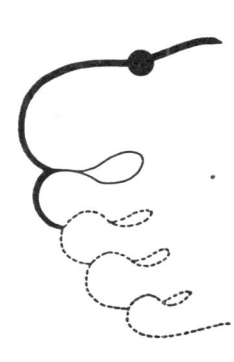

Pineal Gland
-higher, behind pituitary
-both feet
-endocrine system

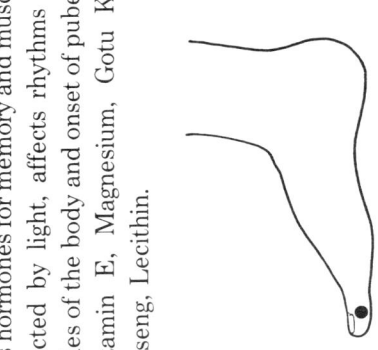

Has hormones for memory and muscles, affected by light, affects rhythms and cycles of the body and onset of puberty. -Vitamin E, Magnesium, Gotu Kola, Ginseng, Lecithin.

Place the side of the index finger (first joint) on the ledge at the side of the big toe, just alongside the base of the nail. Pressure is in towards the big toe then down towards the heel, but there is no movement of the index finger.

Hypothalamus
-in brain, higher above pituitary
-both feet
-nervous system

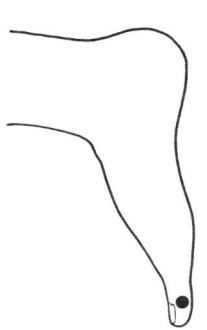

The centre for control of body temperature, of emotions that control heart beat and blood pressure, appetite and fat metabolism, and of sexual reflexes. It greatly influences the activity of certain other endocrine glands as well as a number of specific metabolic functions.

Located halfway between the pituitary reflex and the pineal reflex on the plantar surface of the big toe, slightly higher than both pituitary and pineal reflexes.

7th Cervical
-bump at the back of the base of the neck
-both feet
-structural system

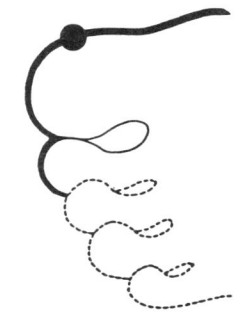

A key point for relaxation from the waist up. If affects the eyes, ears, brain function, and often relieves arms, hands and neck tension.
-Vitamin B Complex, Calcium, Magnesium, Valenan Hops.

Place the side of the index finger (first joint) at the base of the big toe on the arch side (medial) of the foot. Pressure is in towards the big toe and down towards the heel. Don't move index finger up and down or sideways.

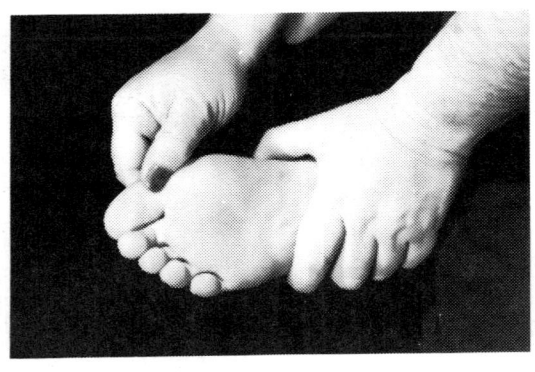

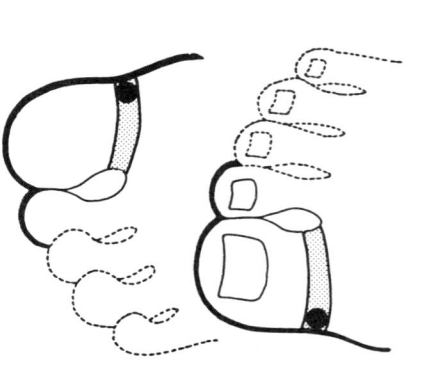

Hook in with the thumb at the base of the big toe on the plantar surface, right near the medial edge of the big toe. The reflex is also located on the dorsal side of the foot, in the same place.

Work these as you would the thyroid. It is within the same reflex.

The reflex is just below the pineal reflex, the little bump on the medial side of the big toe. Use any finger to hook in, around and over the bump.

Thyroid Gland
-across windpipe, in neck
-both feet
-endocrine system

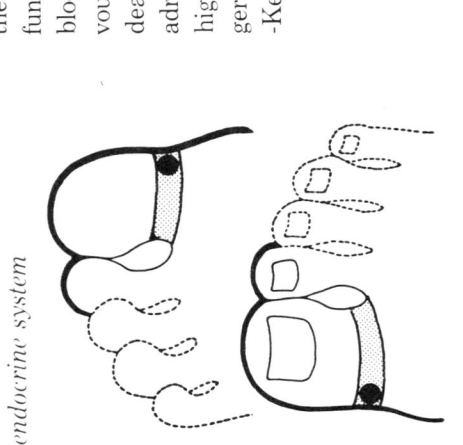

As the thermostat of the body, it regulates metabolism, weight, interacts with the sex glands in emotional and sexual function, and parathyroids to regulate blood calcium level. It affects the nervous system and emotional attitudes, deals with sugar metabolism, stimulates adrenal and sex glands. Is affected in high blood pressure, nervousness, finger tremor, weight problems.
-Kelp, Iodine.

Parathyroid Glands
-imbedded in the thyroid gland
-both feet
-endocrine system

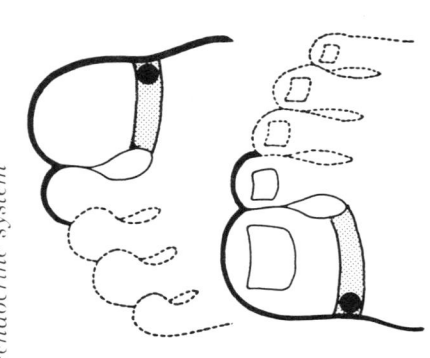
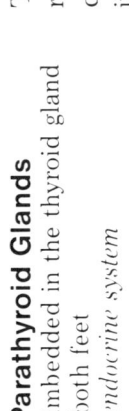

These regulate calcium and phosphorous in the body, affect distribution of calcium by breaking down and reabsorbing it from bones and teeth. Affected in muscle spasms, cramps, sleeplessness, broken bones, arthritis.
-Vitamins C and D, Magnesium, Calcium.

Nose
-head
-both feet
-respiratory system

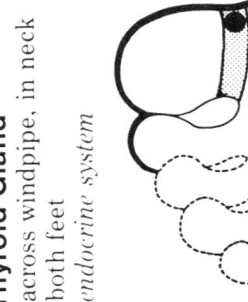
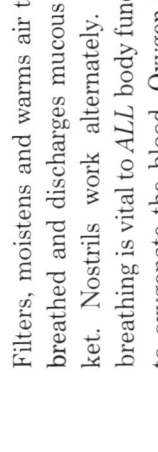

Filters, moistens and warms air that is breathed and discharges mucous blanket. Nostrils work alternately. Deep breathing is vital to *ALL* body functions to oxygenate the blood. Oxygen is the

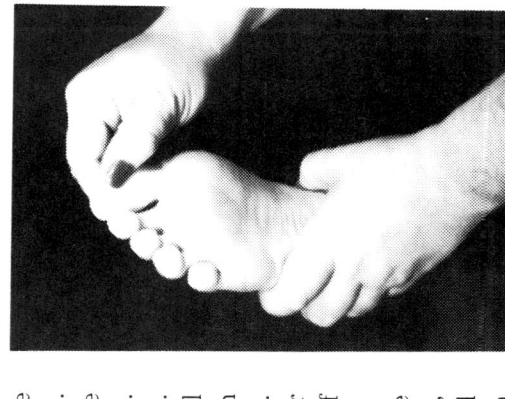
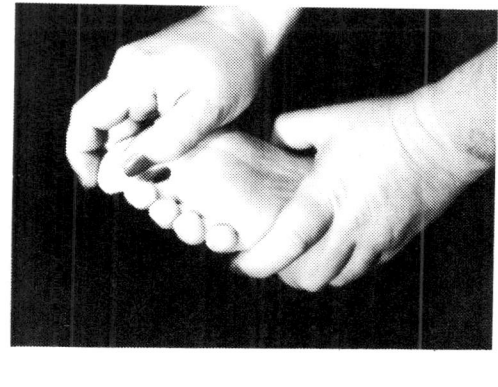

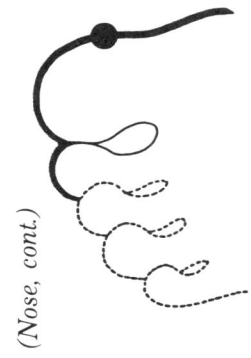

(Nose, cont.)

fuel for energy release. The nose aids the muscles by alternating the function of the nostrils at night causing a person to turn over, eliminating muscular spasms.
-Vitamins A and C, Eucalyptus, Mint, Fenugreek, Sage, Sassafras, Juniper Berries.

Head
-top of the body
-both feet
-structural and nervous system

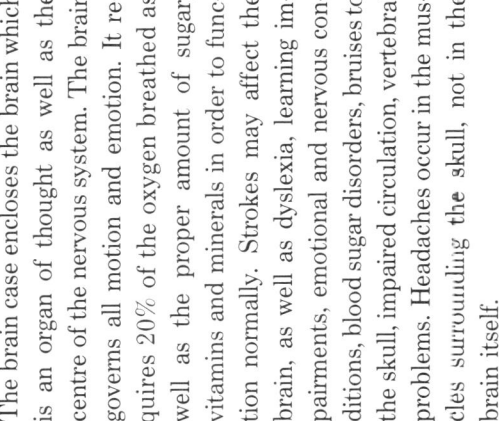

The brain case encloses the brain which is an organ of thought as well as the centre of the nervous system. The brain governs all motion and emotion. It requires 20% of the oxygen breathed as well as the proper amount of sugar, vitamins and minerals in order to function normally. Strokes may affect the brain, as well as dyslexia, learning impairments, emotional and nervous conditions, blood sugar disorders, bruises to the skull, impaired circulation, vertebral problems. Headaches occur in the muscles surrounding the skull, not in the brain itself.
-all Vitamins and Minerals, Lecithin, Gotu Kola.

Walk the thumb over the entire surface of the big toe, up, down and sideways. roll index finger over the very top of the big toe (especially for stroke victims). Inch your nail over the top of the big toe. With your nail, flick the person's toe nail gently. You can repeat the process on the small toes for fine tuning to the head. Gather up all the toes and walk your thumb over the upper edge of all of them, and nail-flick all of them.
NOTE to advanced students: Note the reflexes to the cerebrum, cerebellum, temporal lobe, frontal lobe, base of skull vault. Work each area individually with the thumb, across, up or down the big toe.

Top of Head
Skull
Cerebrum
Cerebellum
Base of Skull
Temporal Lobe

35

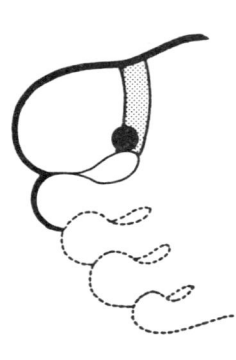

Neck
-between the head and shoulders
-both feet
-structural system
-nervous system
-respiratory system
-digestive system
-endocrine system
-lymphatic system

Holds up the head and is the seat of tension. It has many organs within it, cervicals, thyroid and parathyroid, tonsils, lymph nodes, vocal chords, esophagus, trachea, nerves affecting the arms and hands. It can be the seat of infection. -all Vitamins and Minerals, Valerian, Hops, Mullein, Fenugreek, Slippery Elm.

Walk your thumb along the base of the big toe starting with the plantar surface on the medial side of the foot until you reach the start of the second toe.

Switch to index finger of the opposite hand to walk between the toes, still applying compression to the base of the big toe. The index continues to walk along the dorsal surface of the big toe until you come back to your starting point. Now switch hands to repeat the procedure starting with the thumb of the opposite hand on the inner base of the big toe (lateral side), with your index working the sides and dorsal surfaces. Take tiny steps, 36 steps to go around once is excellent. Work the neck very often, there are many organs within it. (I work the neck for each reflex that is within it.)

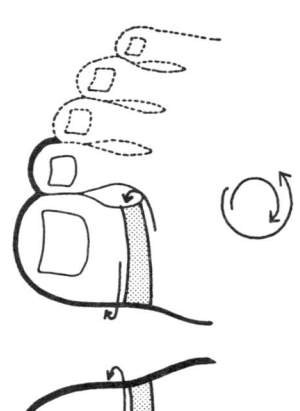

Mastoid Process
-below ear, on lateral sides
-both feet
-structural system

Involved with ear problems, dealing with air circulation and pressure within the ear.

-Vitamin A, B Complex, C, Magnesium.

Hook in with thumb on the edge nearest the second toe, lateral side of the big toe, just above the neck reflex.

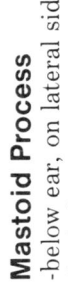

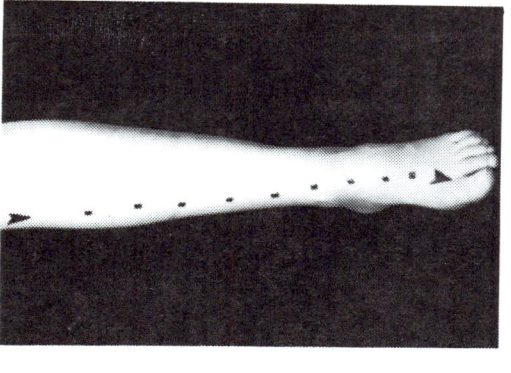
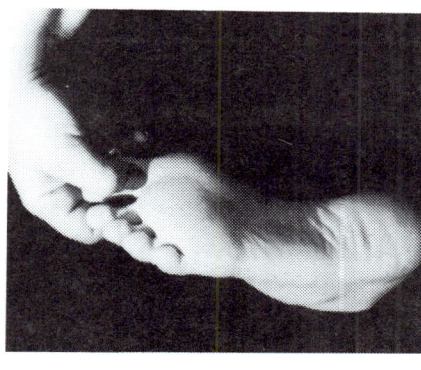

Though the *Drain Plug* reflex is located in the big toe, one starts at the knee using the index finger to trace a line along the bone on the inner edge of the leg, over the dorsal part of the foot, heading straight for the inner corner at the base of the big toe. The thumb hooks in and up on the plantar surface of the inner corner of the base of the big toe. Hook this reflex only *once* on top and only *once* on bottom since it is quite sensitive. Do not work them simultaneously. Use right hand for right foot.

Work these as you work the neck. They are close to the thyroid reflex.

(see Thyroid Gland)

"Drain Plug" Lymphatic Drainage
-base of neck near collar bone
-both feet
-*lymphatic system*

The valve near the neck where the lymph pours into the brachiocephalic veins. Affected in edema and in any swelling or where lymph needs to be drained or properly circulated.

Vitamins A, C, B6, Lecithin, Cider Vinegar, Parsley Tea.

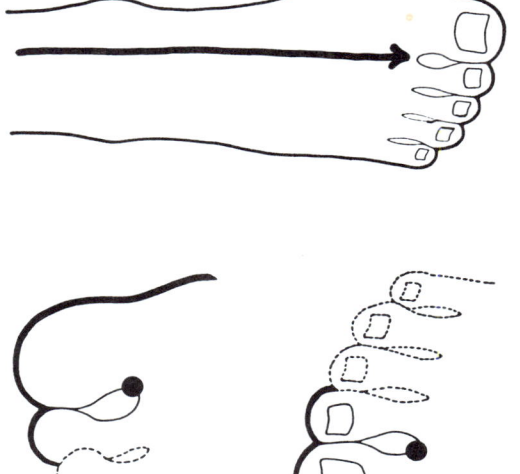

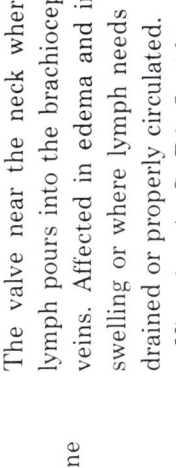

Vocal Chords
-in neck
-both feet
-*respiratory system*

These are mucous-lined ligaments. They are abducted and adducted in breathing and in talking. In breathing they are abducted, or open. In coughing they are closed and then release rapidly, creating the explosive cough. In talking, generally only a thin line of space occurs between the adducted vocal chords, varying somewhat in pitch and volume.

-Vitamins B Complex, C, E.

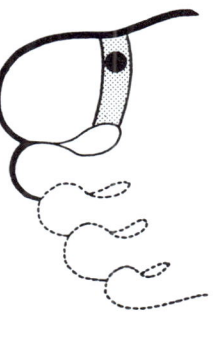

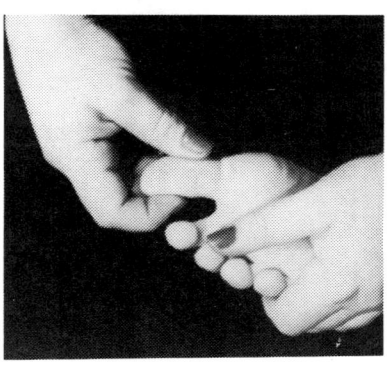

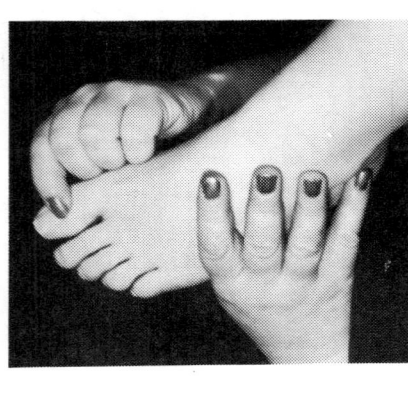

Tonsils
-in the throat naso-pharynx
-both feet
-lymphatic system

The tonsils protect the spine and bronchials from infection by acting as filters. They are large lymph nodes. They affect vaginal discharge and bronchitis particularly when they are removed.
-Vitamin A and C, Chaparral.

Located in the neck reflex. Work the tonsils as you work the neck reflexes; they are centrally located on the plantar surface of the base of the big toe.

(see Neck)

Side of Head
-head and neck
-both feet
-structural system

Affected in headaches and in muscular tension, in TMJ problems and earache.
-Vitamins B Complex, E, Calcium, Magnesium.

With thumb, walk down the lateral side of the big toe from its top to where the big toe joins the ball of the foot. The same reflex, closer to the dorsal side of the big toe is affected in sedation, for insomnia or for relaxation.

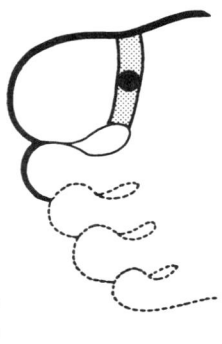

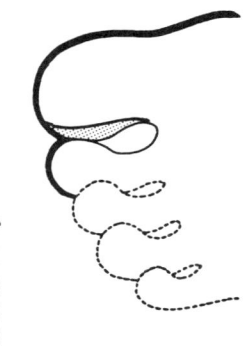

Teeth and Jaw
-mouth/head
-both feet
-structural system
-digestive system

Both aid in digestion by masticating food and mixing it with enzymes to break down starches and sugars. Incorrect placement of teeth or jaw alignment (TMJ) may cause neck problems, shoulder problems, hip problems and sciatica.
-Vitamin C, Calcium, "chewy" foods.

Use index finger to walk just below the nail, above the top joint of each toe. The area closest to the nail represents the upper teeth and upper jaw; the area closest to the joint represents the lower teeth and lower jaw. On the big toe is the reflex to the incisors, second toe, incisor and canine, third toe premolar, fourth toe molar, fifth toe, wisdom tooth.

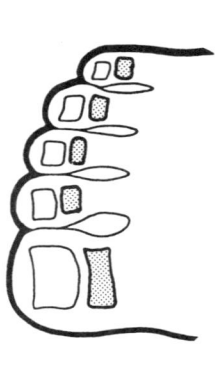

M O S T L Y   T O E S

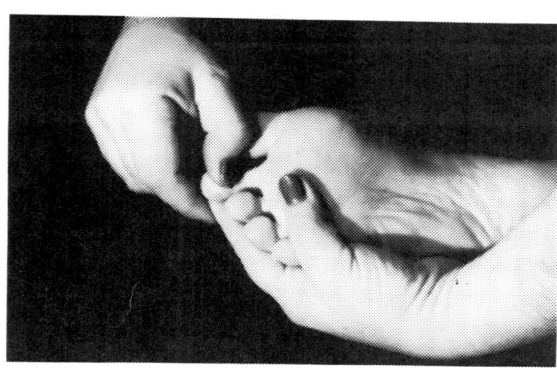

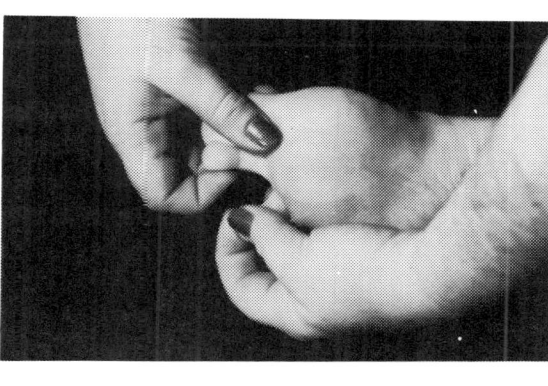

Sinuses
-cheeks, frontal bones, over the eyes, between nose and ears
-both feet
-*respiratory system*

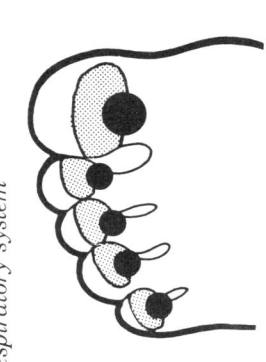

The sinuses moisten and filter the air breathed. They produce lysozyme to destroy foreign objects from the respiratory tract, which forms part of the mucous layer that eliminates foreign particles. Lysozyme acts as an analgesic. They add timbre to the voice and lighten the skull. Should the drainage passages from the sinuses be blocked, inflammation and swelling can occur. Pressure building up within the sinuses causes pain of headache or sinusitis.
-Vitamins A, D and B6, Pantothenic Acid. Eliminate dairy products.

One hand will *totally* cover the entire dorsal surface of *all* the toes, creating both protection from injury from client's own toenails, and a back rest. Place the fingers of the other hand over the back-rest (made by the first hand) leaving the thumb free to hook in and up from under the ball of each toe.
Sinus reflexes will also be found at the back of each toe between toenail and joint.

Eustachian Tube
-from ear to throat
-both feet
-*respiratory system*

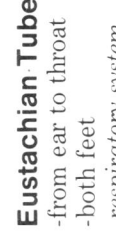 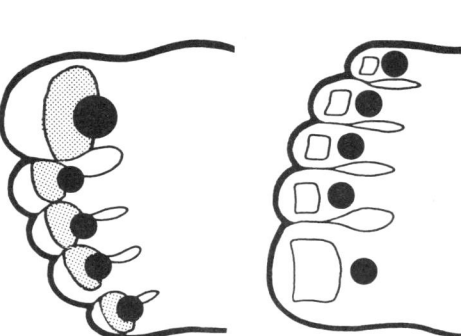

Passes by the ear, removing waste from eyes, ears, sinuses and nasal tract. It also adjusts air pressure in the ear. It is affected in adenoid and ear problems, or when blowing the nose, or when in an airplane. It joins with the naso-pharynx.
-Vitamins A and C, Fenugreek, no dairy products.

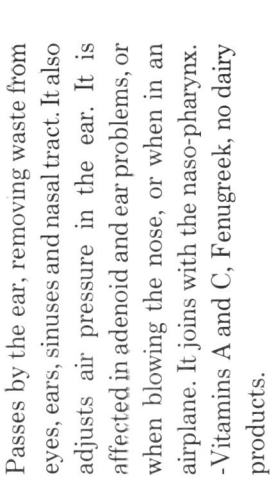

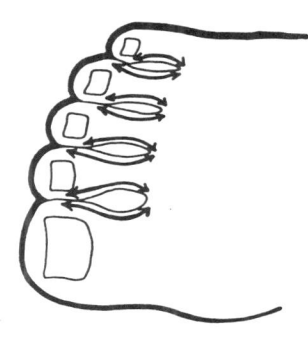

Use your index fingers alternately, to walk down the sides of each toe, on both sides of each toe.

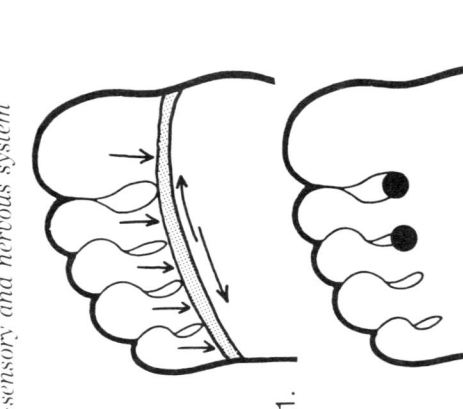
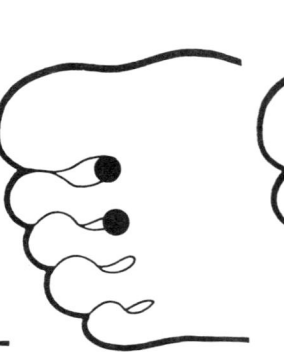
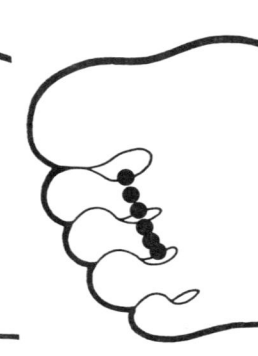
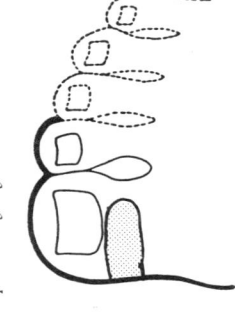

The reflex is on the dorsal surface of the big toe, below the reflex to the teeth and jaw, between the base of the nail and the first joint. Work with your index finger.

Receives the eustachian tube, harbours the adenoids and is sensitive to anything but air. It is involved in the coughing reflex.
-Vitamins A and C, Fenugreek.

Naso-Pharynx
-neck
-both feet
-respiratory system

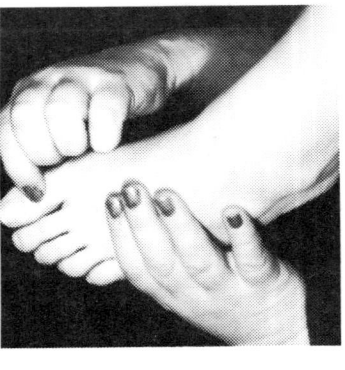

There are three basic reflexes to the eyes.

1) Using the *inner* corner of your thumb, walk across the top of the ball of the foot, just below the toes, pressing down toward the heel. The other hand will press the toes toward the client, exposing the ball of the foot. Work in both directions.

2) Press down with the index finger in the space between the first and second and second and third toes.

3) Squeeze the second joint of the second and third toes, on plantar surface and on each side of the toes.

The eyes are an organ of vision, involved with the kidney, lymph and blood for cleansing and drainage. They are often called the outside view of the brain. Affected by stress, especially shoulder and neck tension. If sensitive, check kidney and coccyx reflexes. Impulses arriving at the visual cortex create a visual image that is spatially oriented and made meaningful with the aid of related association centres. The image received at the occipital lobe is reversed to that actually visualised. Integration of impulses, both visual and memory at the occipital cortex, result in perception of the image as actually seen and interpreted by the brain. The image seen from the right half of each eye goes to the right hemisphere.
-Vitamin A, Eyebright, Parsley, Beets, Carrots.

Eyes
-head
-both feet
-sensory and nervous system

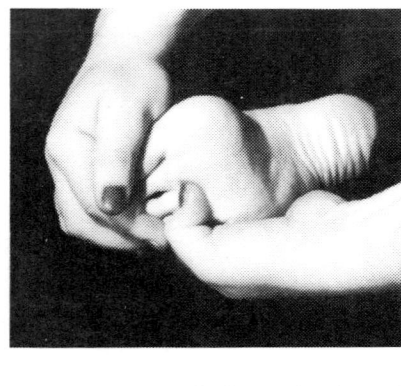
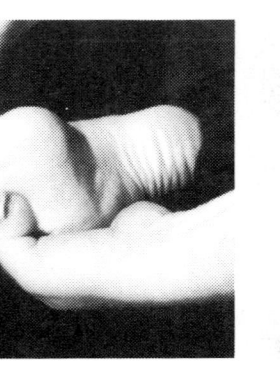
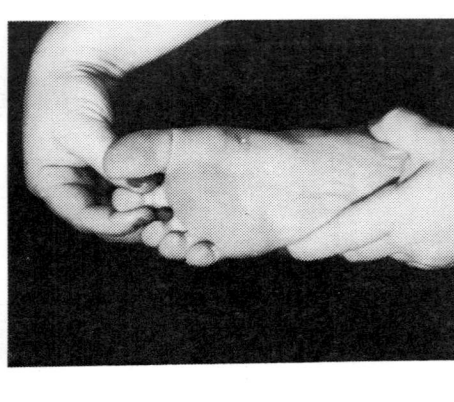
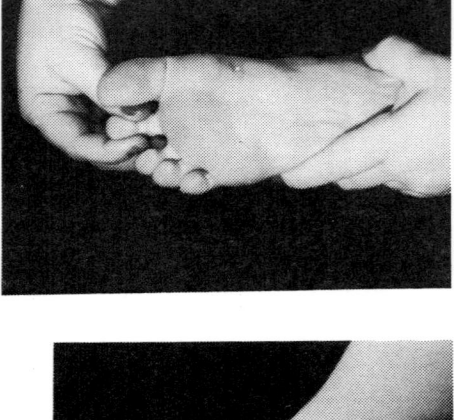

1.

2.

3.

Ears

- side of the head
- both feet
- *sensory and nervous system*

The ear is an organ of sound. The brain has no receptors for sound therefore sound energy must be converted to mechanical energy that can be converted to electro-chemical stimuli, impulses that the brain can deal with. The external ear collects sound waves which are brought to the timpanic membrane. It acts as a resonator, transmits the energy, converting it from sound to mechanical energy. Within the middle ear, the amplitude is increased. Oscillations are created in the cochlear duct, which creates endolymph motion within the duct. This motion bends hair like processes of the receptor cells to the point of discharging electro-chemical impulses which pass on to the cochlear nuclei of the medulla, via the auditory division of Cranial Nerve #8. High pitched sounds come from cochlea stimulation, low pitched sounds come from stimulation of tip of cochlea. Movement of endolymph and bending of hair processes affect and influence eye movement and body position, an adaptive process in spatial orientation. The ear is an organ of balance, it may have an effect on dyslexia. Problems may relate to poor intestinal function, tension in neck and shoulder.

- Vitamin C, Magnesium, Chickweed, no dairy products.

There are three reflexes to the ear.

1) Using the inner corner of your thumb, walk along the top of the ball of the foot, having pressed the toes toward the person you are working on, with the other hand. Thumb pressure is down toward the heel. Walk from both directions. Eye and ear reflexes overlap, as you work one you work the other so always cross the entire top of the ball of the foot.

2) Press down with your index finger in the space between the third, fourth and fifth toes.

3) Squeeze the second joint of the fourth and fifth toes, on both sides.

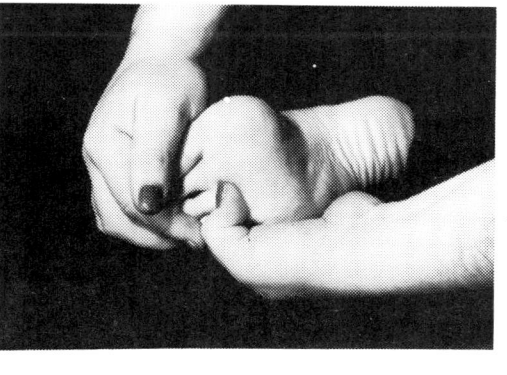
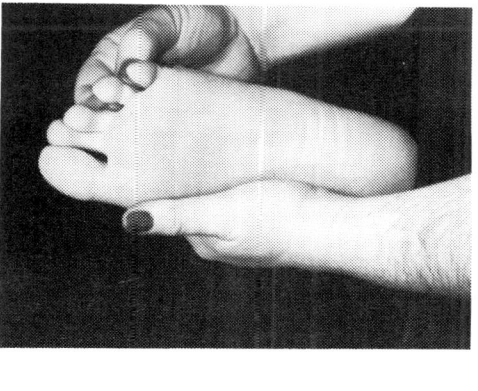
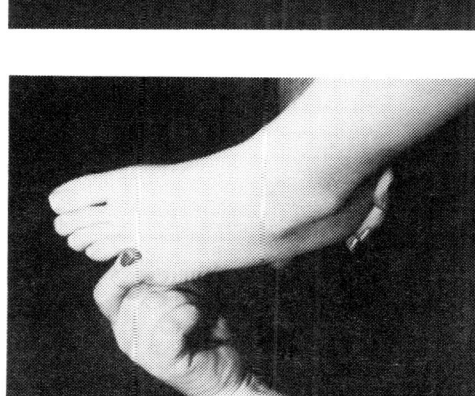

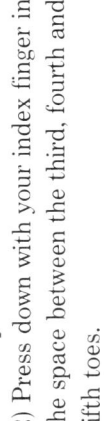
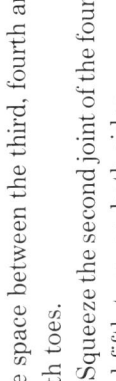
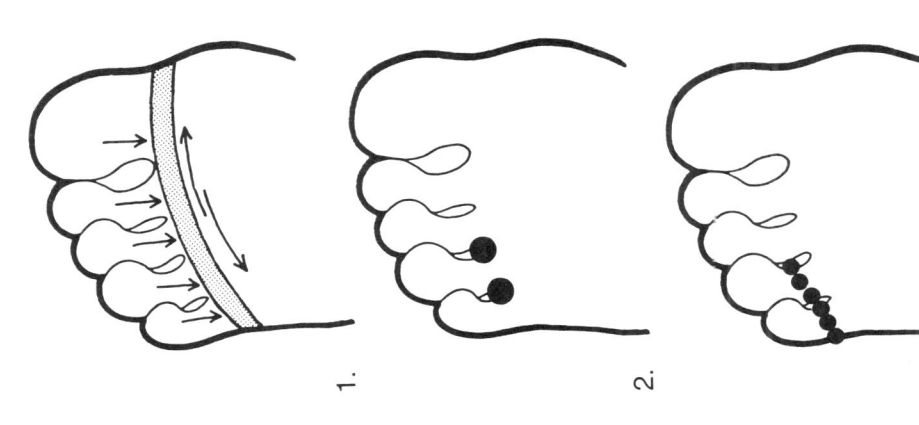

1.

2.

3.

41

MOSTLY IN THE BALL OF THE FOOT

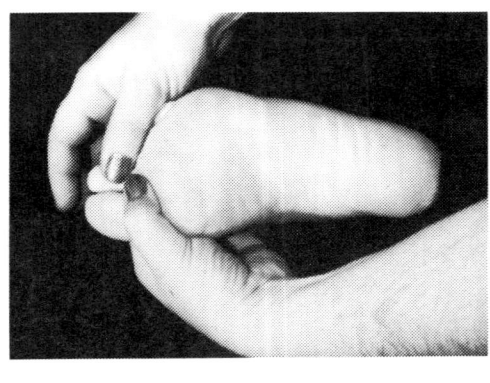

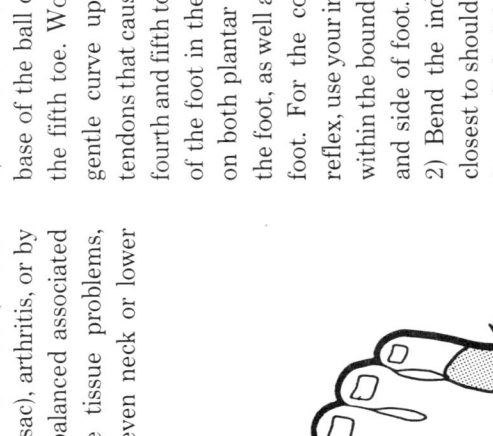

Shoulders
-upper thoracic area
-both feet
-*structural system*

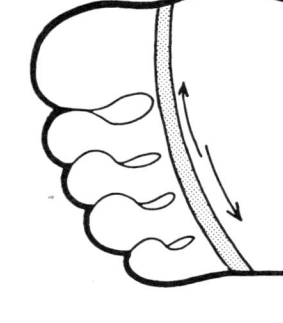

The trapezius muscles often tense causing poor circulation to eyes and ears. The shoulder may affect or be affected by the hips. Shoulder tension is very common. Gall bladder problems may affect the right shoulder, the pancreas may affect the left shoulder.
-Vitamin B Complex, Calcium, Magnesium, Manganese.

Work with the thumb across the top of the ball of the foot, just as you did for the eye/ear reflex, but use the usual outer corner of the thumb, with pressure toward your client. Work from the big toe side to the little toe side, and from the little toe side back to big toe side.

Shoulder Joint
-upper arm attachment
-both feet
-*structural system*

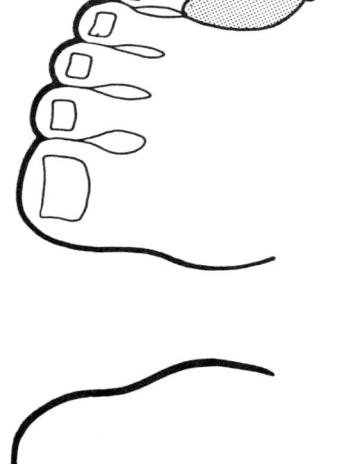

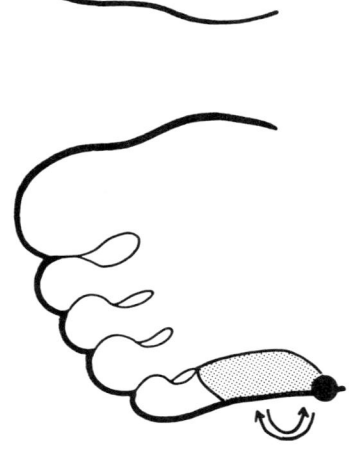

Can be affected in bursitis (inflammation of the bursa sac), arthritis, or by pulled muscles, unbalanced associated muscles, connective tissue problems, muscle strain and even neck or lower arm problems.

1) For the shoulder joint, start at the base of the ball of the foot, underneath the fifth toe. Work from that spot in a gentle curve upward, in between the tendons that cause a groove between the fourth and fifth toes at the top of the ball of the foot in the shoulder reflex. Work on both plantar and dorsal surfaces of the foot, as well as the lateral side of the foot. For the complete shoulder joint reflex, use your index and thumb to work within the boundaries given, top, bottom and side of foot.
2) Bend the index finger of the hand closest to shoulder joint reflex, so that it forms a little *fish hook*. Place the second joint of the *fish hook* directly below the little bone on the side of the foot, below the fifth toe. Anchor your thumb on the ball of the foot and jiggle the *fish hook* up and down.

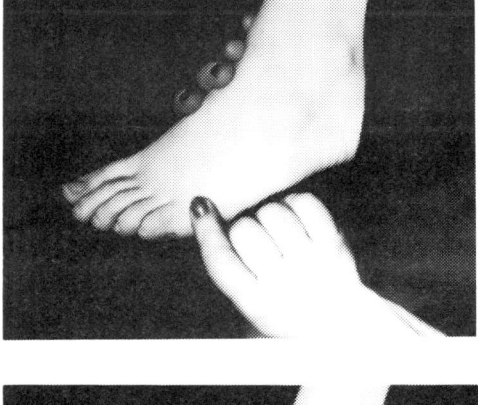

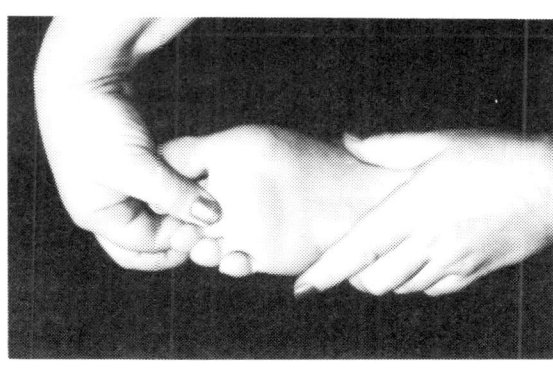

(see above)

3) Place thumb on the ball of the foot below the fifth toe, the index on the dorsal surface below fifth toe, and gently wiggle that part back and forth, completing the shoulder joint reflex.

For the reflex to the head and neck lymph nodes, gently pinch between each of the toes, with index and thumb, on dorsal and plantar surfaces of the foot, where toes join the foot.

Lymph nodes or lymph glands are numerous in the head and neck. They filter toxins from the lymph vessels, protecting the brain, naso-pharynx and throat from infection, manufacturing lymphocytes that destroy harmful substances. Inflamed lymph nodes may notify you of infection in the nose, throat or teeth.
-Vitamins A, C and B6, Cider Vinegar, Fenugreek, Red Clover, Sage, Parsley Tea, Chapparral.

Lymph Nodes of the Head and Neck
-head and throat
-both feet
-lymphatic system

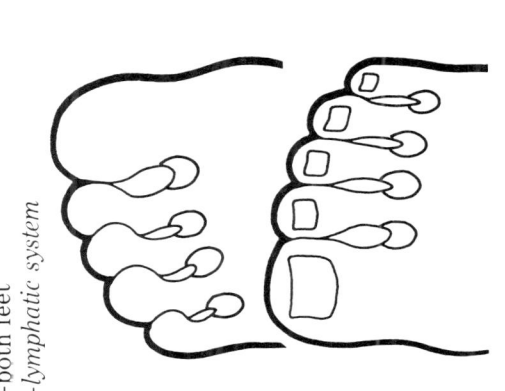

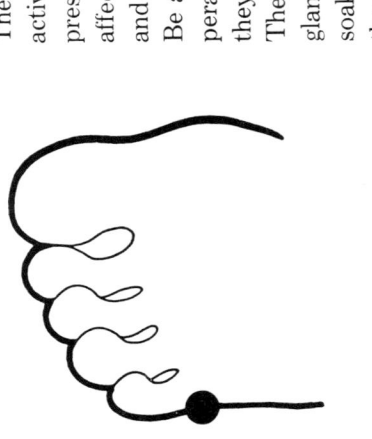

Skin
(organ of elimination)
-covers the entire body
-both feet
-urinary system

As the largest organ of the body the skin throws off three pints, (or two pounds) of waste daily. Tightened or ineffective pores inhibit this action. In a tense person, the adrenal glands order the pores of the skin to close, squeezing out oil. Shiny, oily skin may be a sign of tension.

The skin aids the kidney in eliminating waste, and is often called the third kidney. When an organ of elimination is not functioning properly, the skin helps to eliminate waste. Often, blemishes on the skin point to organs below them that might be malfunctioning, or, they may be caused by hormonal imbalances, as in puberty, or they may be due to improper eating affecting the digestive and eliminative organs.

The skin helps to produce Vitamin D, activates testosterone, regulates blood pressure. It is a sensory organ that affects and is affected by the nervous and emotional nature of the person.

Be aware of skin colour, textures, temperature and changes while you work as they are excellent indicators of tension. There are six miles of ducts to the sweat glands. Sunburn, suntan and over-soaking in hot water tend to deteriorate the skin, which may appeal to skin cancer. The skin affects the organs of elimination, kidney, lung, large intestine. Shingles, a chicken pox virus, shows painfully on the skin, but is an inflammation of nerve endings. Psoriasis is too rapidly formed epidermis. Eczema may be a reaction to sulfur, or foods, or stress.

With the index finger of the nearest hand, apply pressure in and down, with the side of the first joint of the index, to the side base of the pinky toe where it joins the foot. It is located just above the shoulder joint reflex.

(see picture below)

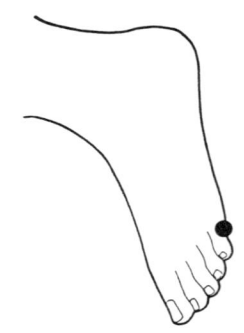

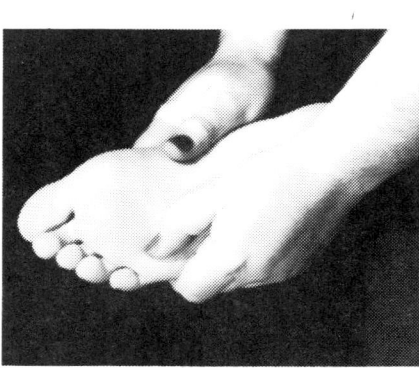

(Skin, cont.)

For dry or oily skin, check the adrenal glands and kidney. Body odour denotes stress and may have its cause in liver malfunction.

-All Vitamins and Herbs that aid the kidney. Perform dry brush massage to aid lymphatics, blood and organs below the skin.

Hook in with your thumb between the fourth and fifth toes, halfway between the top and bottom of the ball of the foot, or midway on the frame of the shoulder joint reflex, plantar side, between the fourth and fifth toes.

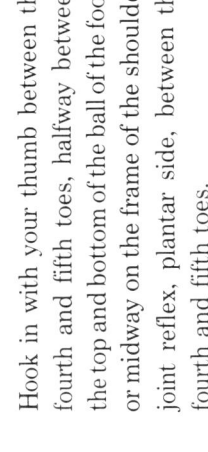

Axillary Lymphatics
-thoracic area in armpit
-both feet
-lymphatic system

There are lymph nodes under the armpits which protect the body from toxins and infections, especially protecting the thoracic cavity. Nodes are generally found in groups, near veins. The lymph nodes enlarge as a signal that an infectious process may be underway.
-Vitamins A, B6 and C, Lecithin, Cider Vinegar, Fenugreek, Red Sage, Parsley, Chapparral.

Use both thumbs alternating across the entire ball of the foot, and, from the top of the ball of the foot to its base. Pay particular attention to the areas between the tendons. You can also walk your thumbs across the foot from medial to lateral side, making sure to completely cover this large area.

Lungs
(organ of elimination)
-thoracic cavity
-both feet
-respiratory system

The lungs eliminate two pounds of waste daily. They are light, spongy tissue, wrapped in individual pleural linings. They help to maintain the acid balance of the blood by blowing out carbon dioxide, and exchanging it for oxygen to fuel the cells. The outside world has easy access to the sterile cavities of the body, via the air/blood interfaces of the lung. The pleural cavity is the space between two layers of pleural lining, and are empty except for a film of fluid that separates the linings, eliminating friction when the lungs move during inspiration and expiration. The base of the lungs

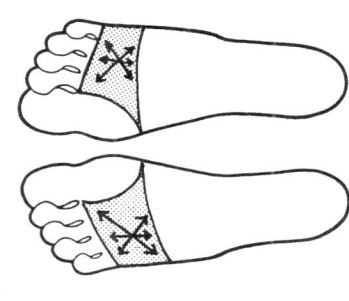

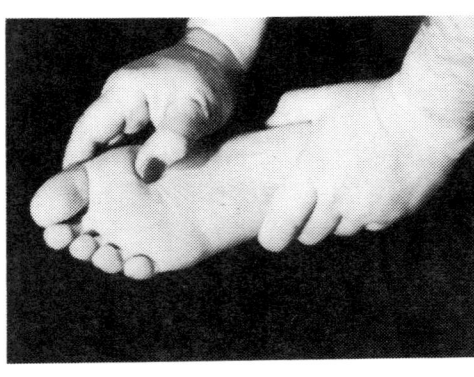

(see picture above)

(Lungs, cont.)

rests on the diaphragm. Deep breathing massages all the organs in the abdominal cavity. Breathing in relates to the thyroid gland, breathing out relates to the parathyroid gland. The lungs are affected in allergies, asthma, bronchitis, pleurisy, pneumonia, and the common cold.
- Vitamins A,B,C,D and E, Fenugreek, Comfrey, Slippery Elm. Calcium, Magnesium.

With your thumb at the base of the ball of the foot on the medial side, walk upwards in the indentation that heads straight between the big toe and the second toe at the top of the ball of the foot.

Esophagus
- centre of thoracic cavity
- both feet
- *digestive system*

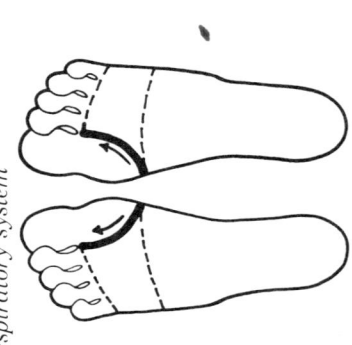

The Esophagus is a tube joining the mouth and stomach. It is affected in stress.
- Vitamin B Complex.

Trachea
- centre of thoracic cavity
- both feet
- *respiratory system*

The trachea begins the lower respiratory conducting tract. It can be felt in the lower neck, just above the sternum, and extends to the level of the second rib attachment to the sternum, or the fourth thoracic vertebrae. There the trachea divides into two main bronchii, one for each lung. It is cleansed by a mucuous layer moved by cilia that line it.
- Vitamin A, C,D and E, Fenugreek, Slippery Elm, Comfrey.

With your thumb at the base of the ball of the foot, on the medial side, walk upwards in the indentation that heads straight between the big toe and the second toe at the top of the ball of the foot. Same as the *esophagus* reflex.

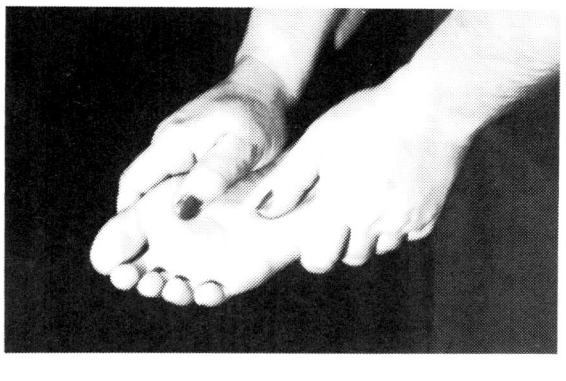

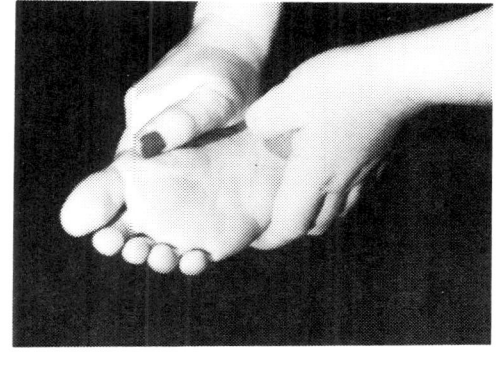

Find the widest portion of the *bunion* area. Now with your thumb move to the trachea reflex. Hook in sideways, toward the *bunion* right in the centre of the trachea reflex. Generally, you will note a lumpiness here, that is quite distinguishable and sensitive.

Work gently with the thumb over the plantar edge of the ball of the foot on the medial side, right by the *bunion* area. Also found on the dorsal surface below the big toe on the *bunion bump*. Use your index on the dorsal surface.

Thymus Gland
-thoracic cavity above heart, over the trachea, under the sternum
-both feet
-lymphatic and endocrine system

The thymus is the chief of the body's defense system. It trains and regulates antibodies in the body's effort to fight all invaders. It is affected by and affects stress, all diseases, and allergies. The thymus inhibits the pituitary growth hormone, but is affected by the same growth hormone for its own size. It increases the number of stem cells in bone marrow, stimulates lymphocytes and inhibits neuro-muscular transmission. It is often referred to as an endocrine gland. In allergy it is over-reacting to what it considers a dangerous substance. This occurs in transplants of organs as well. Under stress conditions, it shrinks too much to effectively combat disease, so that disease may often accompany stress.

-Vitamin A and B, Thymus glandular substance, Golden Seal, Chapparal.

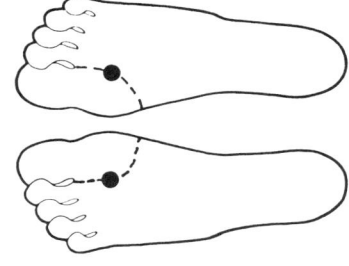

Sternum
-thoracic cavity
-both feet
-structural system

Located in the front of the body, it forms the frontal attachment for the upper seven ribs. The Xyphoid process is its lowest point. It helps in protecting the lungs, trachea, esophagus, heart, thymus gland, and maintenance of proper rib structure and therefore upper back.
-Calcium, Phosphorous.

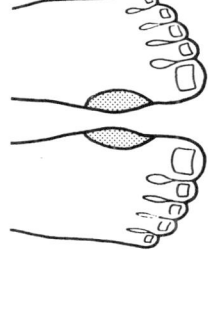

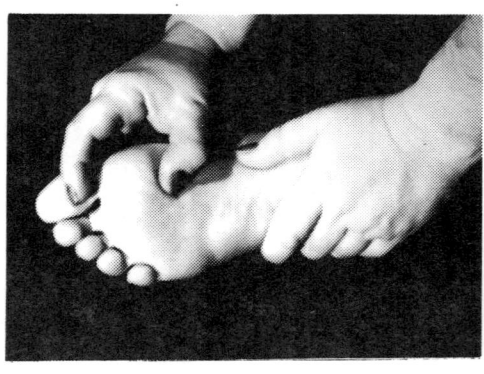

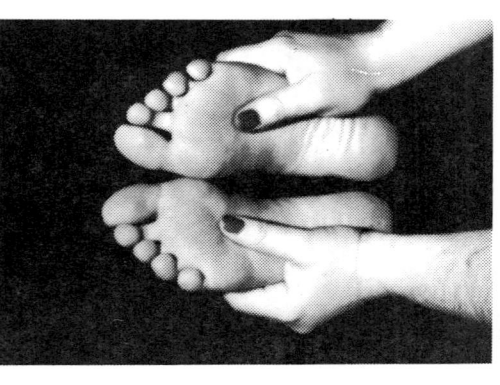

Work the thumbs in both directions, at the base of the ball of the foot, with pressure upwards toward the bony structure of the ball of the foot. Make sure your steps are small so that you reach all parts of the diaphragm reflex, from medial to lateral edge and back again.

The diaphragm separates the chest cavity from the abdominal cavity. It contracts downwards, flattening to pull air into the lung, and relaxes, curving upward, to push air out. It regulates breathing by contracting and expanding. It is affected in asthma, blood pressure problems, hiccups, nervousness, emotional trauma and hiatus hernia. It is a seat of relaxation.

- Vitamin B and C, Calcium, Magnesium.

Diaphragm
- thoracic cavity and upper abdominal cavity
- both feet
- *respiratory system*

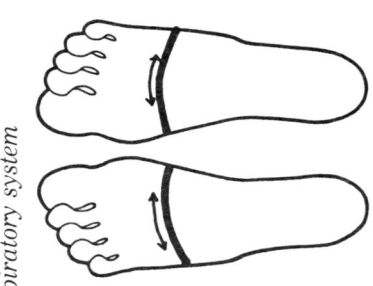

Place both thumbs simultaneously on both feet, in the centre of the diaphragm reflex, at the base of the ball of the foot, in the little niche that just fits your thumb. Hold the reflex lightly and gently, applying no pressure. Have your client breathe deeply. This reflex is used during the colour breathing, the affirmation stroke and for solar plexus breathing at the end of a session. It relaxes the system, lowers blood pressure. Start a session holding the solar plexus, end it with Solar Plexus Breathing. (*See Chapter 12.*) Return to this reflex when you encounter pain in another reflex.

The solar plexus is your main reflex for relaxation. Twelve pairs of nerves extend to all parts of the body. Excellent for ticklish or overly sensitive feet at the start of a session and also to end it with lasting relaxation. It relaxes the body through the para-sympathetic system. It brings circulation to the extremities, feet, hands and head. When worked, a person's hands or feet may perspire.

Solar Plexus
- abdominal cavity between sternum and navel
- both feet
- *nervous system*

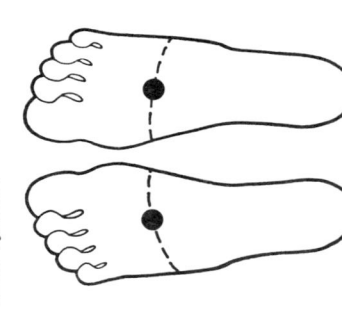

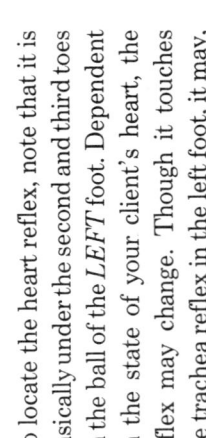

(*see picture below*)

To locate the heart reflex, note that it is basically under the second and third toes on the ball of the *LEFT* foot. Dependent on the state of your client's heart, the reflex may change. Though it touches the trachea reflex in the left foot, it may,

The adult human heart is an extremely efficient muscular pump, designed to contract 42 million times per year and eject 700 thousand gallons of blood in that time. Although the design of this pump is simple, the control mechanism

Heart
- thoracic cavity, left of centre
- left foot in healthy heart
- right foot in complications
- *circulatory system*

48

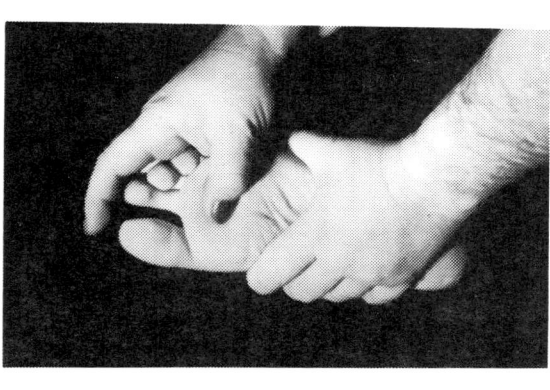

(Heart, cont.)

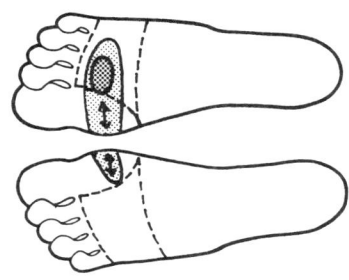

for heart rate and cardiac output is exquisitely sensitive and elaborate. Blood entering the heart is first sent to the lung to oxygenate it. This oxygenated blood returns to the heart and is then pumped out of it and throughout the entire system, to bring nutrients and oxygen to each cell and to remove wastes from each cell. The heart contains its own intricate system of blood vessels to supply itself with nutrients. 20% of your calcium intake is used by the heart. Specialized tissue, called juntional tissue, possesses the property of rhythmical impulse formation and conductivity. One of these junctions is called the *pacemaker*.

The adrenal glands may cause the heart to beat more rapidly when there is need. The cardio-vascular regulatory centre in the medulla oblongata, in the brain, controls heart rate. This centre is stimulated by higher centres in the brain, primarily located in the frontal lobes, where emotional disturbances of anger, fear, excitement are rapidly transmitted through the hypothalmus. The primary control of heart rate is through the vagus nerve. When stimulated there is an inhibitory effect, slowing the heart rate and lowering blood pressure. As blood is pumped through the arteries and returned through the veins it exerts a certain amount of pressure. Arterial pressure is a product of the cardiac output and the peripheral resistance to the blood flow that exists in the arterial system at any given moment. Blood pressure is con-

if enlarged, reach the trachea/thymus reflex in the right foot, and extend to the shoulder joint reflex in the left foot. Use your thumbs to work the reflex in all directions, and along its periphery. If the reflex to the solar plexus is very sensitive check the heart reflex.

An oval hard round callous on the left foot only may pertain to the heart. Remember that you are *NEVER* to diagnose when you are working on the foot. If the reflex to the heart is sensitive, and if the person requests it, you may tell your client that there is congestion or tension in the body. If you are very concerned and with good cause, you might ask "When did you have your last medical check-up?" and suggest that it is time for another one. *AND THAT IS ALL!* Do not mention heart problems, heart attacks or high blood pressure. A client is very suggestible and you may provoke the problem that you were trying to avoid.

(continued on next page)

(Heart, cont.)

stantly in flux.

-Vitamin B,C and E, Calcium, Magnesium, Potassium, Iron, Chromium, Selenium, Lecithin, Hawthorne Berry, Cayenne, Garlic.

U P P E R   D O R S A L   O F   F O O T

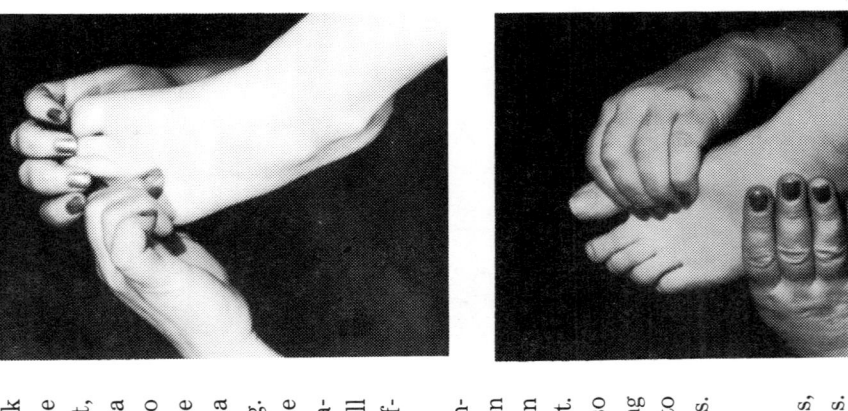

The bronchials enter the lung like an upside-down tree, separating from the trachea into one branch for each lung, then dividing into bronchioles, and re-dividing, until they become very tiny *twigs* at the end of which are alveoli, (air sacs) which resemble a broccoli head. In the alveoli, the exchange of oxygen and carbon dioxide occurs, as each blood cell trades off its waste for life-giving oxygen. Cilia line the entire respiratory tract, moving a mucous blanket upwards into the throat and mouth where it is either expectorated or swallowed. The mucous traps dust, bacteria etc. and cleanses the lungs, bronchials and throat.

-Vitamin A and C, Calcium Flouride, Fenugreek, Comfrey, Slippery Elm.

' On the dorsal portion of the foot, alternate your index finger to walk between the tendons that go to the toes, from where the toes join the foot, to where the tendons meet. To get a better effect, one hand can be used to separate the toes, the thumb on the ball of the foot pushing up on the area that the other hand's index is working. This allows you to reach well into the reflex between the tendons. Alternating your fingers again accesses all parts since each index hooks at a different angle.

BRONCHITIS REFLEX Place four fingers between 1st and 2nd toes, thumb on ball of foot. Perform a milking action on the big toe as if you expected it to squirt. Keep your hands firmly on the skin, so that you do not chafe it. This milking action can be performed on all the toes to benefit the bronchials and back muscles. Use the most convenient hand.

To work the reflex to the back muscles, one of your hands will separate two toes. With the index finger of the other hand, hook in between the tendons on the dorsal surface of the foot, from the toes to where the tendons join and stop your

Bronchials
-thoracic cavity, within lungs
-both feet
-*respiratory system*

Back Muscles
-thoracic area, in the back
-both feet
-*structural system*

The back muscles hold the spine in place and must be equally balanced on both sides for proper funtioning of the spine and the nerves emanating from it. They are affected in whiplash and sports injuries as well as overwork or faulty

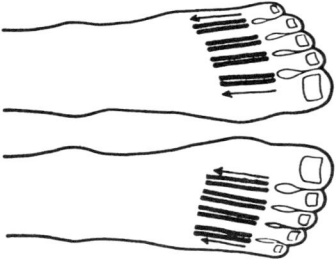

50

(see above pictures)

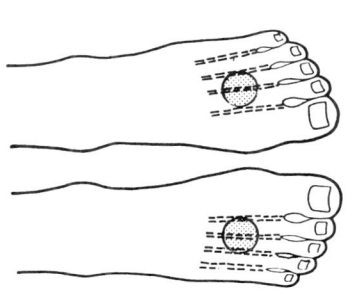

finger's progress. Switch hands so that the index of the other hand is accessing a different angle. Work between each toe with each index. Note where there is tightness, sometimes between two tendons, sometimes near the toes, sometimes near the junction of the tendons. Tension here may denote tension in that part of the back to which it reflects.
WHIPLASH REFLEX is the same as the bronchitis reflex. Milk the big toe. Pretend that you are milking an upside down cow. Milk the other toes as well. Note that the reflex to the back muscles is identical to the reflex for the bronchials.

The breast reflex is between the 2nd and 3rd toes on the dorsal surface of the foot in the reflex to the bronchials. Use your index fingers to work this area well especially in lactation or in case of cysts.

(Back Muscles, cont.)

movements. They affect and are affected by neck, shoulder and even hip or low back problems and definitely in stress. They work in groups along the back, but are also in league with muscles in the front of the body in order to rotate, flex, extend, adduct or abduct arms, legs, hips, shoulders or head. They are the seat of tension along with the neck and shoulder muscles.
-Vitamin B Complex, Calcium, Magnesium, Manganese, Zinc.

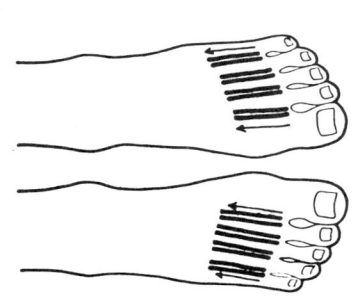

Breast
-thoracic area
-both feet
-reproductive and lymphatic system

The breast is composed of various glands and ducts packed in fatty tissue, along with nerves, blood and lymphatic vessels. Just before the ducts in the breast converge to form the nipple, they dilate to form lactiferous sinuses, which function as milk reservoirs during lactation. The lymphatic vessels in the breast drain the fat portion of the milk, produced during lactation and are also a vehicle for the transfer of infected material from the breasts to more distant parts. The axillary lymphatics protect the breasts. Milk production is the result of the action of many hormones, influencing the gland's cells. The letdown and excretion of milk results from a neuro-endocrine reflex mechanism, imitiated by the suckling baby at the nipple.
-Dang Quei, Nucleoproteins, RNA, Chlorophyll.

51

UPPER ARCH PORTION OF FOOT

Adrenal Glands
-abdominal cavity above kidney
-both feet
-*endocrine system*

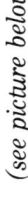

The adrenal glands are like two different glands encapsulated as one, the cortex and the medulla outer and inner portions. The medulla secretes and releases epinephrine, which stimulates the metabolic rate and the breakdown and mobilisation of starch, lipids resulting in more available energy. It elicits the fight/flight reaction in response to life threatening situations and increased nervous system activity. It causes dilated pupils, increased blood supply to the muscles, blood shunted away from skin and gastrointestinal tract to more critical areas, increased respiration rate, increased heart rate and force of contraction. The medulla is highly involved in stress and reactions to stress, and is controlled primarily by the sympathetic nervous system.

The synthesis of epinephrine requires the cortical hormone, cortisone.

The adrenal cortex secretes hormones dealing with the fluid-electrolyte balance, such as aldosterone and other mineralocorticoids. They affect the salt/potassium ratio in the system. Other cortex hormones affect carbohydrate metabolism, such as cortisol and other glucocorticoids and low level sex hormones. ACTH from the anterior lobe of the pituitary gland stimulates the secretion of glucocorticoids. Aldosterone is secreted in response to certain enzymes in the blood. These hormones play roles involving all aspects of protein, carbohydrate, electrolyte and water metabolism.

(see picture below)

1. On the right foot, place your left hand across the entire waist reflex to locate the waistpoint on the medial side of the foot in the plantar region. With your right hand, draw an imaginary line between the waistpoint and the base of the ball of the foot, nearest the arch and below the big toe. Now cut that imaginary line in half. That halfpoint is the adrenal reflex. It is on the medial side of the tendon that goes from the big toe down to the heel. (That tendon may be located by pressing the client's big toe towards her, exposing the tendon.) Use your right thumb for the adrenal reflex in the right foot. If you then place the remaining four fingers over the entire ankle, while the thumb is on the adrenal reflex, the angle that you use when you hook your thumb will be perfect for this reflex.

2. On the other side of the tendon, just above the kidney and slightly down from reflex number 1, hook in with thumb. Note right adrenal is slightly lower than left adrenal.

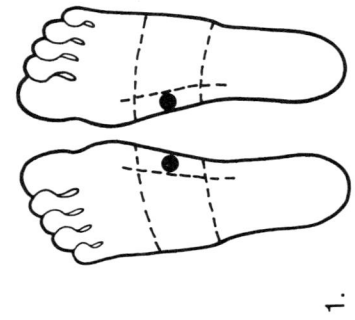

1.

2.

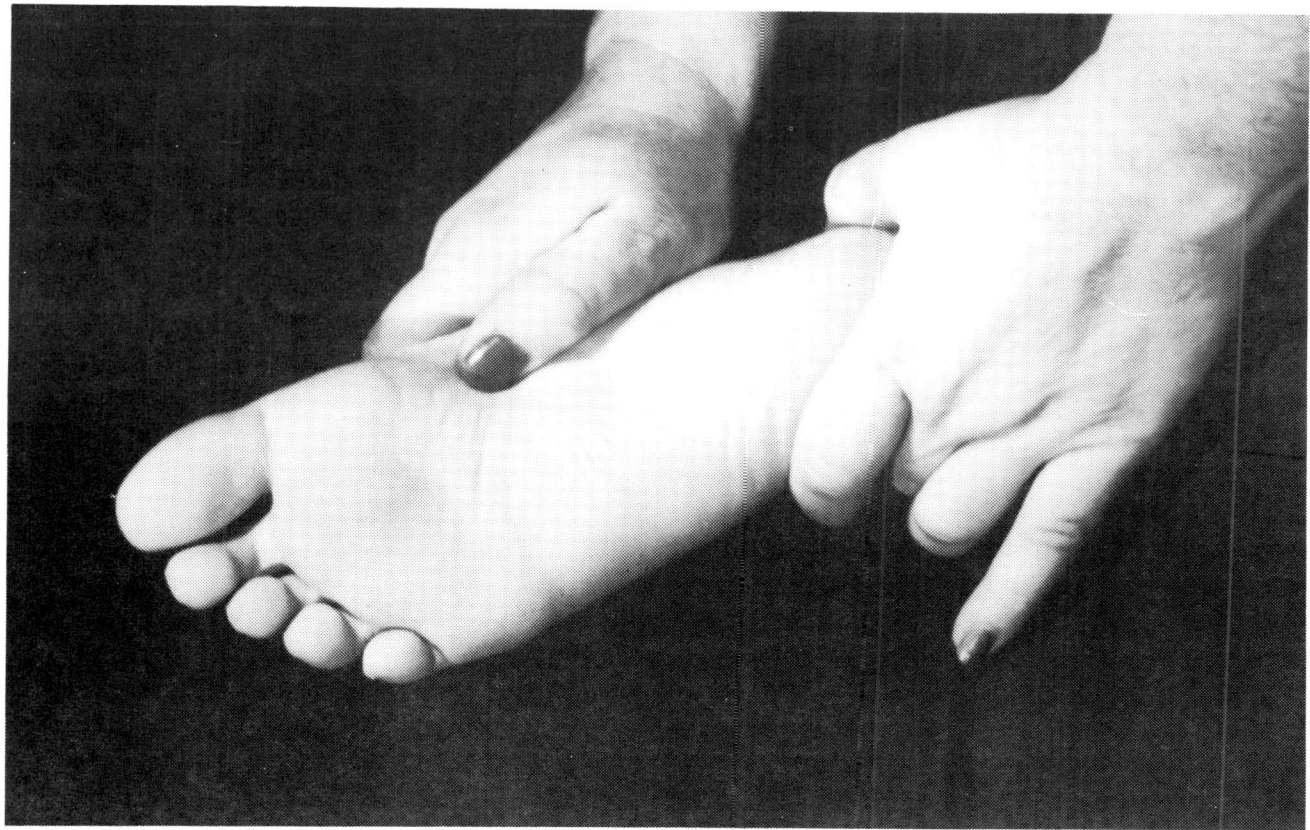

(Adrenal Glands, cont.)

Thus the adrenal cortex is necessary for life. In Addisons disease, there is an inability to withstand stress, no appetite, weakness and other symptoms.

Overactivity of the adrenal cortex, involving sex hormones, causes masculinization of females and precocious development of secondary sex characteristics in prepubescent males.

Cortisone has a variety of metabolic effects in all tissues, inhibits the incorporation of amino acids into the cells, may deal with the anti-inflammatory action of this steroid.

The innermost cortical zone is responsible for adrenal secretion of androgens and estrogens. It is affected by the pituitary gland. Substantial amounts of sex steroids may be of adrenal origin. The adrenal glands may be involved with low blood pressure, high blood pressure, the defense system, allergies, arthritis, asthma, heart action, skin and muscle tone, and are always affected by stress. Having over 50 functions, the adrenals are involved with the health and maintenance of the system and require extra attention.

-All Vitamins and Minerals, particularly B Complex, Vitamin C and Calcium.

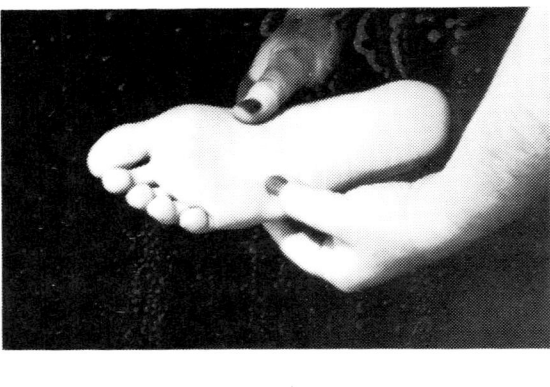

The reflex to the liver will be found on the right foot. Alternate the thumbs to really cover this large reflex, and come at it from all directions, work from the base of the ball of the foot to the waist of the foot, and from the edge of the foot below the fifth toe, (below the ball of the foot) to the second toe. The upper third of the reflex will extend to the medial edge of the foot, while the lower two thirds of the reflex end below the second toe. If you alternate thumbs as you work you will not tire from working this extensive reflex. Cover the entire area well and be aware of its sensitivity in dis-ease or when medication is being taken.

Liver
-abdominal cavity, right side, below diaphragm
-right foot only
-*digestive system*

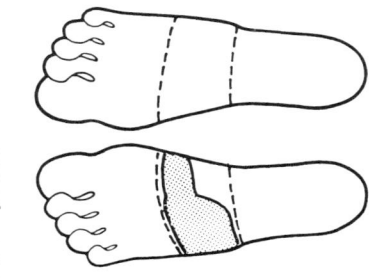

The liver is the filter and detoxifier of the body with over 500 other functions. It is often called the *King of the Glands.* Its functions range from blood clotting and blood thinning to the digestion of foods. It affects migraines, indigestion, blood cholesterol, allergies to food, constipation, bile flow, blood sugar, varicose veins, hemorrhoids. It changes old blood cells sent to it from the spleen, into bile, which it sends to the gall bladder for storage and dispersal. If the gall bladder or spleen are removed the liver will take on their function. Since the liver is the filter and detoxifier of the body it will be affected by any drugs, medications consumed, and its reflex may be sensitive. Also, since it has so many functions and 1,000 enzymes, if there is anything wrong with the body, the liver will be involved. The liver can regenerate itself if a portion is removed provided the diet is exemplary and no medication is taken.
-Vitamin A,B,C and D, Lecithin, Cayenne, Lemon Juice.

Gall Bladder
-abdominal cavity, within the lower lobe of the liver; right side
-right foot only
-*digestive system*

The gall bladder stores bile for proper breakdown of fats and carbohydrates, neutralizes the acidity of chyme from the stomach, as it goes to the duodenum. The bile leaves the gall bladder through the cystic duct, which merges with the common bile duct, and enters the duodenum. The gall bladder contracts in response to gastro-intestinal hormones and the vagus nerves, and

To work the gall bladder reflex, form a "C" with your left hand, as if you were about to lift a cup with a thick handle. Arrange the "C" so that your index is between the 4th and 5th toes on the dorsal surface in between the tendons. The thumb is between the 4th and 5th toes on the ball of the foot, plantar surface. Slide your hand down until the joining tendons on the dorsum of the

(see picture below)

54

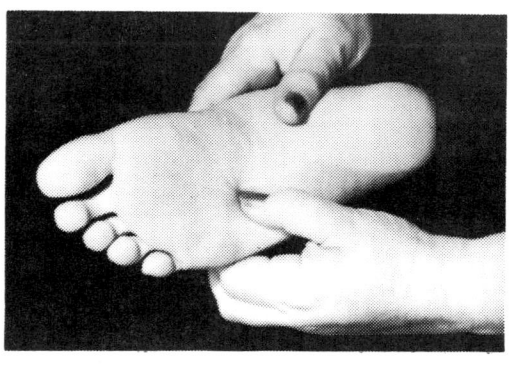

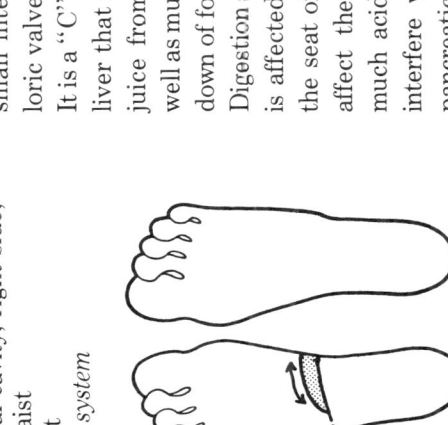

(Gall Bladder, cont.)

bile is directed to the duodenum. The yellowish bile colour is due to the presence of pigments (bilirubin). It renders the ingested fats more soluble in water, to aid in digestion. Bile breaks up masses of fat into small globules. Gall stones may hamper the function of the gall bladder, by blocking the common bile duct, causing bile to back up into the gall bladder, also the back-up of pancreatic juice (which shares the common bile duct) back into the pancreas. Gall stones are crystalized bile salts and cholesterol.

-Vitamin A, Lecithin, Lemon Juice.

foot stop your index finger. Move your thumb down, so that it still lies between the 4th and 5th toes, but is below the ball of the foot within the liver reflex. Now, pinch both index and thumb together. In some people this reflex is found between the 3rd and 4th toes, so check with each individual for the most effective reflex.

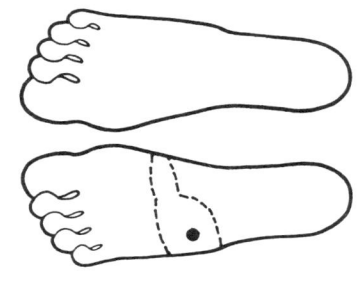

Duodenum
-abdominal cavity, right side, above waist
-right foot
-*digestive system*

The duodenum is the first part of the small intestine, starting after the pyloric valve, at the base of the stomach. It is a "C" shaped structure, below the liver that receives bile and pancreatic juice from the common bile duct, as well as mucous. Within its walls, break-down of food is acted upon by enzymes. Digestion and assimilation begin here. It is affected by stress and may often be the seat of duodenal ulcers. Stress can affect the pyloric valve, allowing too much acid from the stomach, or, may interfere with the timing of bile and pancreatic juices which may irritate the unlined duodenum leaving it open to ulceration.

-Vitamin B Complex, Magnesium, Raw Cabbage/Potatoe Juice (for ulcers).

The duodenum reflex, on the right foot, is a gentle curve, above the waist, from the medial edge to below the 4th toe where it is on the waist. Work the boundary with your thumb and its inside with alternating thumbs to reach all parts of the reflex.

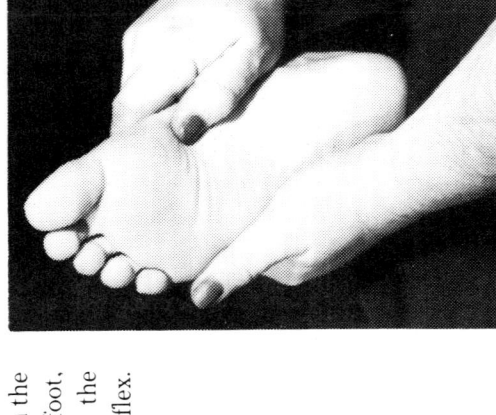

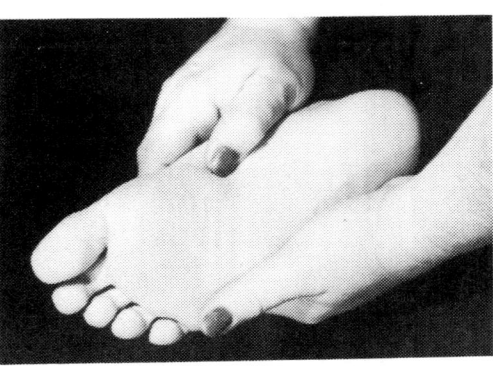

(see picture below)

Hiatus Hernia
-abdominal cavity, top of stomach at diaphragm
-right foot only
-*digestive system*

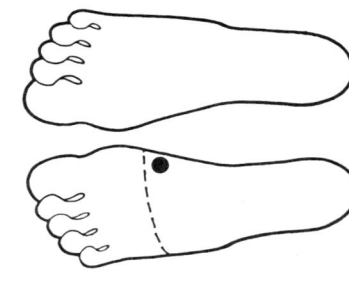

A hiatus hernia may occur when a portion of the stomach is squeezed into the thoracic cavity, through a hole in the diaphragm, by the base of the esophagus. It causes exquisite pain after eating or when bending forward.

The hiatus hernia reflex is found on the right foot, below the ball of the foot, underneath the big toe, between the adrenal reflex and the diaphragm reflex. Hook in with your right thumb.

Pylorus (Pyloric Valve)
-abdominal cavity, base of stomach
-right foot only
-*digestive system*

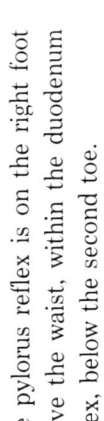

The pylorus regulates the flow of chyme, allowing only small amounts of it to enter the duodenum at any given time. It prevents the back-up of bile into the stomach. Bile salts are damaging to the stomach lining.

The pylorus reflex is on the right foot above the waist, within the duodenum reflex, below the second toe.

Stomach
-abdominal cavity, below diaphragm, left side
-covered by ribs
-left foot only
-*digestive system*

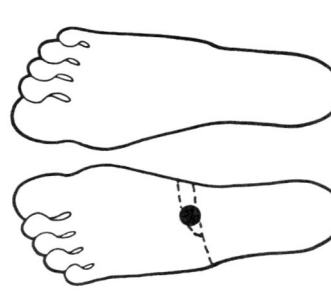

The stomach is the first part of the gastro-intestinal tract, suspended from the liver and diaphragm, and may rest on bladder or uterus after a full meal. It stores ingested food, preparing it for eventual treatment by the small intestine. Waves of contractions, along

For the stomach reflex, on the left foot only, start with the left thumb, walking just below the diaphragm reflex, following the same curve as the bony structure of the base of the ball of the foot but below it. The thumb will curve gently as does the diaphragm reflex, until you

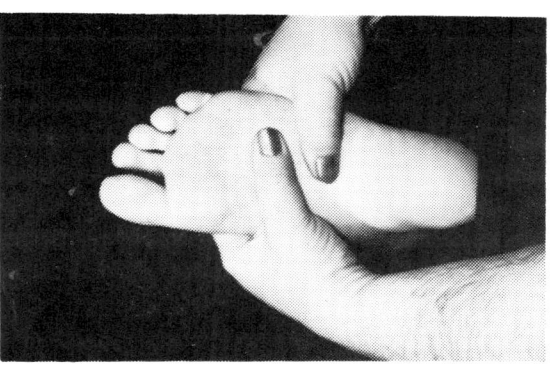

(Stomach, cont.)

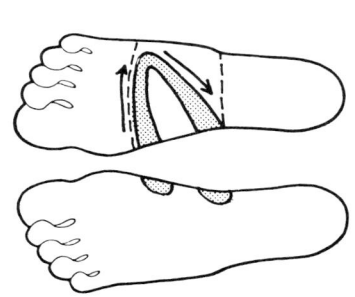

smooth muscles, create an agitator action in the gastric pits, similar to that of a washing machine. As a result, long chain molecules are broken down into smaller components. Protein is specifically broken down into smaller units by the enzyme, pepsin, which is activated by hydrochloric acid, and secreted by parietal cells. Pepsin and other enzymes make up gastric juices, that would have an erosive effect on the surface mucosa if it weren't for the mucous secreted by the mucous cells. Very little food absorption goes on at the stomach level. The stomach secretes a sugar protein compound, (intrinsic factor) which influences the absorption of Vitamin B12 from the small intestine, which is vital for red blood corpuscles. Gastro-intestinal hormones influence stomach activity, as does the vagus nerve. The stomach affects and is affected by emotional stress, and, though highly acidic, many gastric complaints stem from too little acid and too few digestive enzymes. Food is broken down layer by layer then passed on through the pyloric valve. Basically the stomach breaks down proteins into smaller chains to allow further breakdown and absorption in the small intestine.

-Vitamin B Complex, Magnesium, Comfrey, Cayenne, Potato and Cabbage Juice (raw), Lemon or Cider Vinegar in water, Pepsin, Digestive Enzymes, Papaya, Betaine Hydrochloride.

reach the spot between the 4th and 5th toes. Now, switch to the right thumb, which will actually be on the spleen reflex, when it is placed next the the left thumb. The right thumb will now head downwards a few steps then describe a gentle curve, downwards and back across the foot toward the medial edge at the waist point. Only the bottom part of the stomach reflex touches the waist, at the medial side. The stomach is always worked in this direction, left thumb from arch to pinky toe side, right thumb from pinky toe side sloping toward arch side ending at the waist. The untouched portion of the area you have worked is the pancreas reflex.

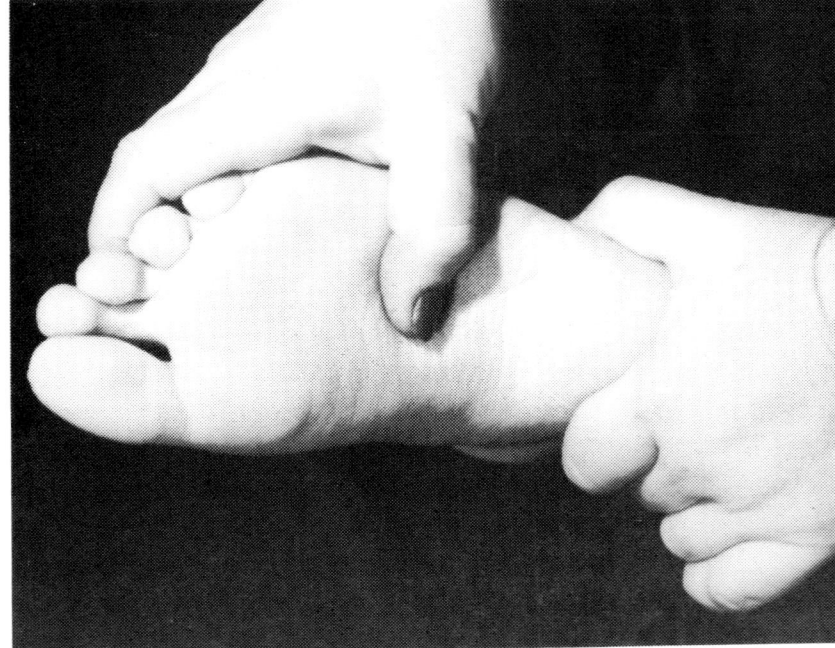

(see picture below)

Pancreas

-abdominal cavity behind stomach, mostly on left side, Islets of Langerhans on right side
-mostly left foot
-in hypo/hyper glycemia work also on right foot
-endocrine system
-exocrine gland/digestive system

The pancreas is a dual gland, both endocrine and exocrine in function. The endocrine function of the pancreas deals with insulin production, important in the sugar balance of the individual, allowing simple sugar, glucose, a body fuel, to be utilized effectively. Insulin is secreted by the Islets of Langerhans, specialized cells in the pancreas. Insulin facilitates glucose transport into cells, together with potassium. It increases glycogenesis and lowers blood concentration of glucose. Insulin acts on the muscles to increase incorporation of amino acids and formation of protein. Insulin also acts on fat cells to increase glucose entry and oxidation and to lead to lipogenesis. Insulin increases the glycogen formation. Secretion of insulin is stimulated by an increase in plasma glucose and by parasympathetic nervous activity. It is inhibited by sympathetic nervous activity, and by epinephrine. Glucagon increases glycogen breakdown and glycogenolysis in the liver, which stimulates glucose uptake into the muscle. It inhibits amino acid incorporation into the muscles. This hormone decreases serum calcium and increases cardiac contracting ability. Secretion of glucagon is stimulated by hypoglycemia and by sympathetic nervous activity, inhibited by the parasympathetic system. In other words the endocrine function of the pancreas deals with diabetes (hyperglycemia) and low blood sugar (hypoglycemia).

The exocrine function of the pancreas helps in the breakdown and assimilation

The pancreas reflex, on the left foot, occupies the, as yet, untouched centre of the stomach reflex. Start with your left thumb on or near the adrenal reflex and walk it in a light upward slant, toward the spleen reflex. The pancreas reflex ends at the spleen reflex, between the 4th and 5th toes, below the ball of the foot. It can be worked from either direction, with either thumb. There is a small portion of the pancreas reflex on the right foot, just below the adrenal gland reflex, below the big toe (1st zone).

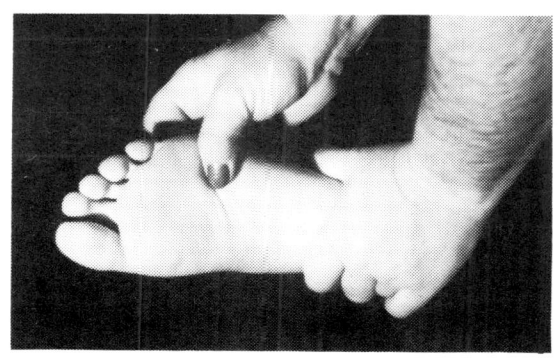

On the left foot only, use the same "C" technique as you used to find the gall bladder reflex in the right foot, but now make a "C" with the right thumb and index, place the index between the tendons of the 4th and 5th toes on the dorsal surface, and the thumb between 4th and 5th toes on the ball of the foot. Slide thumb and index down until the tendons' junction stops the index finger, and the thumb is below the ball of the foot, between 4th and 5th toes. Pinch index and thumb together.

(Pancreas, cont.)

of fats, carbohydrates and proteins through pancreatic juices that enter the duodenum via the common bile duct. If the duct is clogged with gall stones, pancreatic juices may back up into the pancreas to irritate and inflame it.

-Vitamin B Complex, Rice Polishings, Horsetail Tea, Oat Straw Tea. Limit sugar, caffeine, alcohol. Limit sweet fruit, bananas, raisins, prunes etc.

NOTE: Hypoglycemia often goes hand in hand with Candida Albicans whose many symptoms include bloating after meals, depression, energy loss and basically deals with an over abundance of yeast in the system. Requires professional advice.

The spleen is the largest lymphoid organ. It forms blood cells, filters injurious substances from the blood stream, aids the liver in filtering and "housekeeping", removes iron from old blood cells, stores that iron for future use, then sends the useless dead blood cell to the liver, where it is turned into green bile. It stores bile pigment, bilirubin, and is very active in the immune system of the body. It is affected in blood diseases (malaria, leukemia, hemophilia) and in anemia.

The spleen affects bacteria and parasites in the body. It also is involved in lowering blood pressure, along with the diaphragm and solar plexus reflexes.

-Vitamin A and C, Iron, Cayenne, Garlic, Onion, Parsley Tea, Beets, Carrots, Watercress, Nasturtium, Cranberry.

Spleen
-abdominal cavity behind stomach
left side
-left foot only
-*lymphatic system*

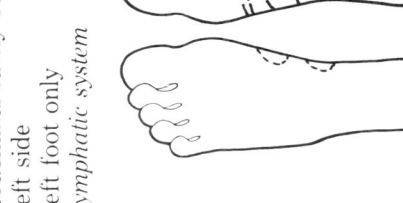

LOWER ARCH OF THE FOOT

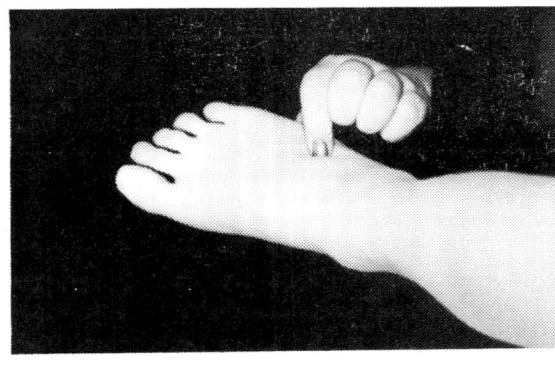

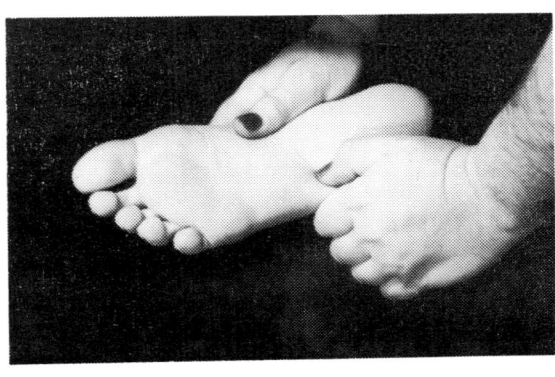

Appendix
-lower abdominal cavity, right side
-right foot only
-*digestive system*

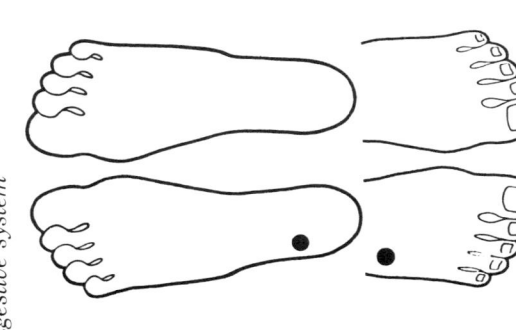

The appendix is a blind pouch at the beginning of the large intestine, just below the ileo-cecal valve. It may be involved in the antibody and the mucous function of the body. Since it has no muscular bands it cannot eliminate waste that backs up into it. This waste may irritate, inflame and infect the appendix. If the appendix ruptures, the person is in grave danger as toxic waste invades the peritoneal cavity. If you suspect appendicitis, make sure to obtain medical help immediately.
-Bowel Cleansing Herbs.

1. Press the left thumb just above the heel, between the 4th and 5th toes. Hook in deeply, with presure exerted toward the lateral edge of the foot. Since the reflex is deep, you may need to press the right thumb over the left to obtain more pressure.

2. This reflex is located one finger joint from the base of the fifth metatarsal, on the edge of the cuboid and calcineum bones, and under the fifth metatarsal, both on dorsal and plantar surfaces.

Ileo-cecal Valve
-lower abdominal cavity, jointure of ilium and cecum
-right foot only
-*digestive system*

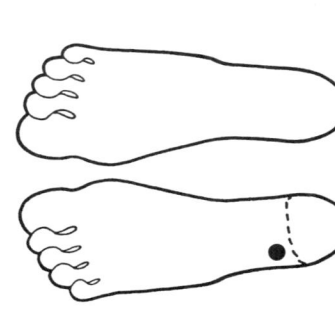

The ileo-cecal valve is the valve that allows waste to leave the small intestine, to enter the large intestine without allowing waste to back-up into the small bowel and the peritoneal cavity. It is also the mucous plug of the body, and is involved in cases of too much or too little mucous in the rest of the system. It is affected in sinusitis, ear infection, bronchitis, dry or flowing nose or eyes, constipation, diarrhea, etc...
-Bowel Cleansing Herbs, Vitamin A, Fenugreek.

The ileo-cecal valve and the appendix share reflex # 1 above. Place your left thumb just above the heel between the 4th and 5th toes. Hook in deeply, with pressure exerted toward the lateral edge of the foot. Since the reflex is deep, place right thumb over hooked left thumb to make deeper and more exact contact.

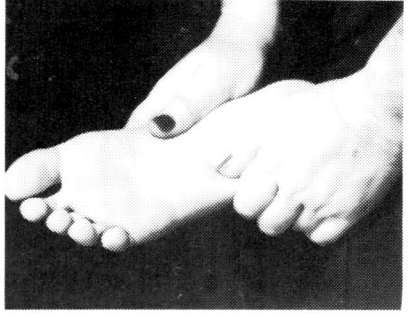
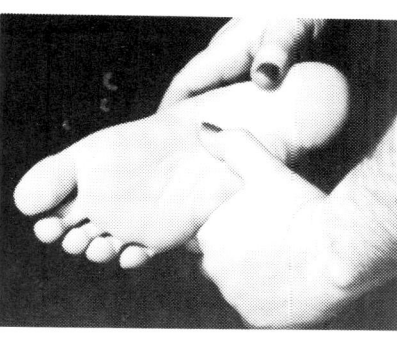
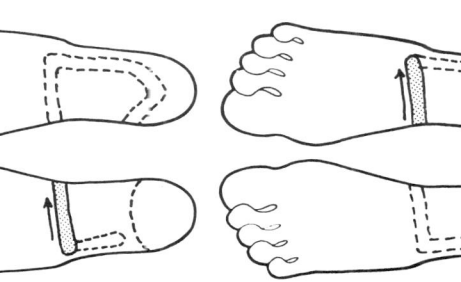

Large Intestine (organ of elimination)

-lower abdominal cavity, surrounds the small intestine
-both feet different
-*digestive system*

The large intestine is an organ of elimination, excreting at least two pounds of waste daily. It is controlled by muscular bands that push waste along through a process called peristalsis. To function properly the muscles need good tone or fecal matter will not be adequately moved and the colon may prolapse, may form diverticules (balloon-like projections which trap waste, becoming inflamed in diverticulitis), and become coated with thickened waste particles that impede elimination.

The appendix is at its beginning. The ileo-cecal valve is located near it. The ascending colon rises to the waist, below the liver, and curves at the hepatic flexure to become the transverse colon, turns down at the splenic flexure, below the spleen, to become the descending colon, turns upward to become the sigmoid flexure, where feces are retained until eliminated, then downward into the rectum and anus.

The function of the large intestine is to reabsorb fluid, vitamins and minerals from the waste and return them to the system by passing them through the portal and hepatic veins to be filtered by the liver before being re-released. Its function is to convey waste in a semi solid state. Bacteria in the colon are both *friendly* and *unfriendly*, some manufacture vitamins and break down carbohydrates and proteins producing amines, acids and gasses; some are eliminated, others are purified by the liver. The waste products of the *unfriendly* bacteria, are a

Reflex to the Ascending Colon and half Transverse Colon. Right foot only - ONE DIRECTION

Walk your left thumb up from the ileocecal reflex to the waist remaining in the 4th zone. This is the ascending colon reflex. At the waist is the hepatic flexure reflex. Turn your left thumb so that it can walk along the waistline of the foot to the arch side (medial side). This represents the right half of the transverse colon. This completes the large intestine reflex on the *right foot*.

Half Transverse Colon, Splenic Flexure, Descending Colon, Sigmoid Flexure, Rectum, Anus. Left foot only - ONE DIRECTION

Continue with the left thumb walking on the waistline of the foot, but, as you reach the third toe, give a slight lift to the colon reflex to raise it just a tad above the waist, until you reach the 4th zone. This is the reflex to the splenic flexure. Now, switch to the right thumb to walk down the 4th zone to the start of the heel. This is the descending colon reflex. At the heel, the reflex to the sigmoid flexure begins. With your right thumb, take a 45 degree angle to get to the centre of the heel, then, angle 45 degrees back up but to the medial edge of the heel so that you have formed a wide *V* shape at the heel. (The sigmoid reflex is deep so make your hooking and walking steps quite deep and firm.) Now for the rectum reflex, slide your thumb around the outside of the heel (not on the walking surface) medial side, so that the entire inner side

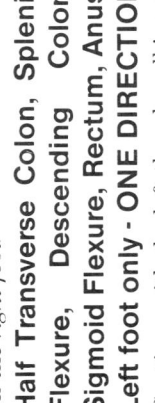
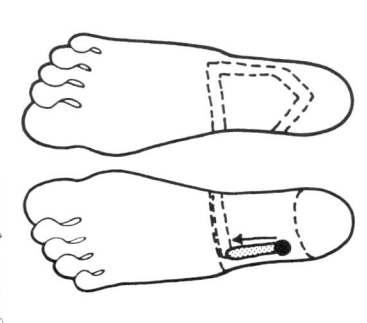
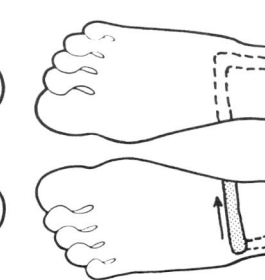

(continued over)

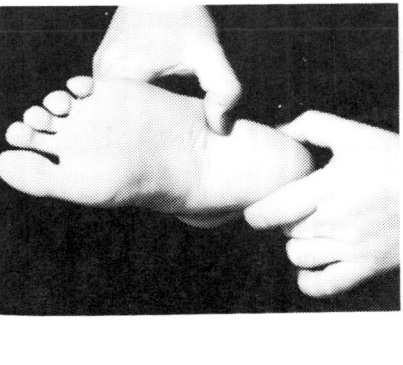 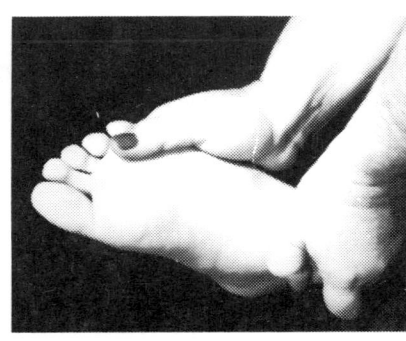 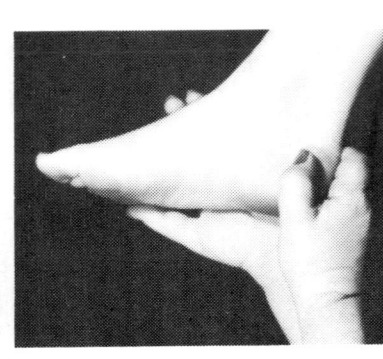

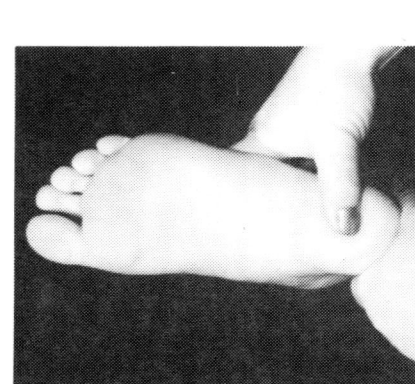

of the first joint of your thumb is pressing into the medial heel edge of the foot. Use your left thumb over the right thumb for added pressure.

Now walk from medial edge of heel where your thumb is lying toward the back of the heel, bypassing the bladder reflex, and below the uterus/prostate reflex for the anal canal reflex.

Remember to work only in the direction specified to obtain the best effect and to avoid colon irritation.

variety of gasses and histamines, both of which can cause discomfort if they are excessive. (Too much histamine can affect allergic reactions to bee stings etc, too much gas can cause great pressure in the colon, pressing upward with force enough to even move the heart.)

The large intestine affects the respiratory system, mucous disorders, diverticulitis, colitis, bowel diseases, constipation (too long a time in the bowel, too little mucous, no muscle tone, too dry), diarrhea (waste moves too fast, too little fluid removed, much vitamin/mineral loss, dehydration). Constipation may stem from a prolapsed colon, prostate problem, low back pain, and may in turn affect the entire system. Arthritis, ear problems, even cancer may stem from a malfuntioning large intestine. Some practitioners of different methodologies believe that *ALL* diseases stem from the malfunctioning lower bowel.

-Vitamin A,B,C,D, and E, Psyllium Seeds, Bran, Fiber Foods, Garlic, Cayenne, Bowel Cleansing Herbs.

(Large Intestine, cont.)

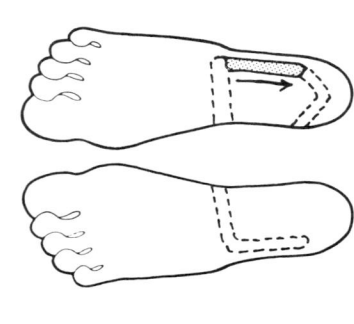 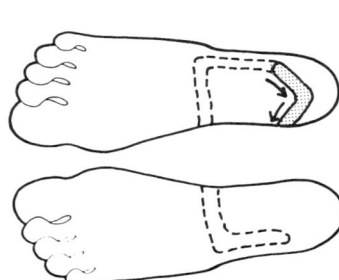

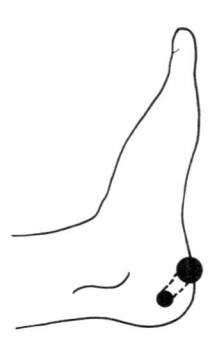

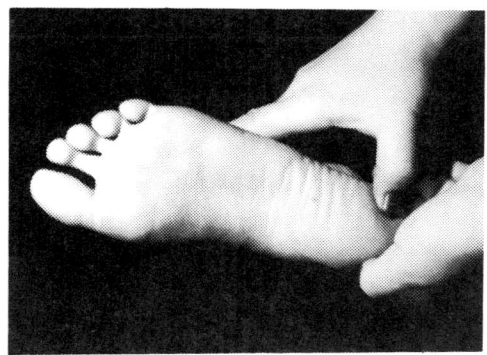

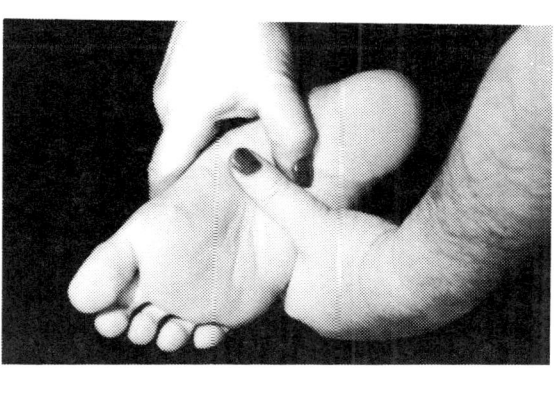

Hemorrhoids
-rectum
-both feet
-*digestive system*

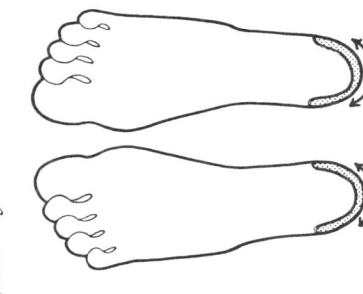

Hemorrhoids are varicose veins in the rectum caused by too much pressure against the rectum, incorrect elimination habits, or childbirth. Varicose veins are an effect of the liver's function so be sure to work the liver reflex.

For hemorrhoids walk along the curve of the edge of the entire heel on both feet. Hook in deeply. This same reflex can be used for acute back or hip pain.

Small Intestine
-lower abdominal cavity within the confines of the large intestine
-both feet
-*digestive system*

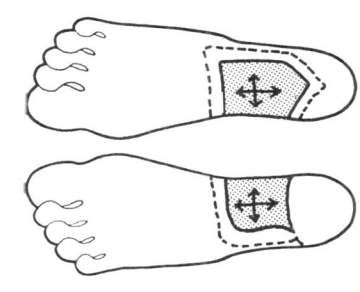

The small intestine is an organ of assimilation, modifying foods that leave the stomach, and processing them in small amounts at a time. Its 20 feet are coiled up. In the duodenum (first part), food that passes the pyloric valve is alkalinised and is assaulted by enzymatic action. In the jejunum and ilium (second and third parts) foods are further changed into absorbent particles, amino acids, glycerol, fatty acids and glucose. The jejunum and ilium contain hair-like villi that separate useful bits from waste and extend the absorbing surface of the intestine and assimilate useful nutrients, assimilating through blood and lymph capillaries in and around the villi, sending them to the liver for filtering and processing.

The small intestine is affected by stress. Strong emotions may halt the almost constant movements it makes as it shifts food particles through its length, leaving

Whereas the duodenum has its reflex above the waist, the jejunum and ilium reflexes are below the waist, within the boundaries set by the large intestine reflex. Work with either or both thumbs, in all directions.

On the left foot a portion of the small intestine reflex will be in the heel, where the sigmoid flexure has dipped down into the heel.

Work the small intestine reflex extremely well as this area is vital to the system.

Note any fleshiness on the dorsal surface of the foot; it may point to intestinal disturbances.

Keep one thumb over the transverse colon so that you do not work it in the opposite direction by mistake.

(continued over)

63

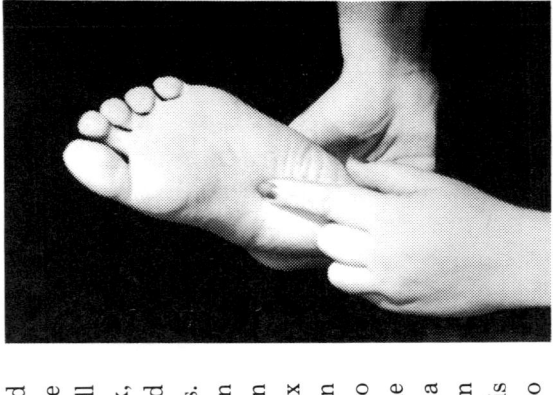

(Small Intestine, cont.)

undigested, un-broken down particles as waste to be passed through the ileo-cecal valve into the large intestine for removal. Certain vitamins are made in the small and large intestine in the presence of bile such as vitamin K (for blood clotting) certain B vitamins and vitamin D.

-All Vitamins (particularly B Complex) and all Minerals, Cayenne, Yarrow, Fennel, Chaparral, Garlic, Black Walnut.

Kidney (organ of elimination)
-abdominal cavity between waist and 12th rib, each side of spine
-both feet
-urinary system

The kidney filters the blood, preserving the proper balance of salts and water in the blood and body, recycling useful material back into the bloodstream, eliminating waste of about 3 pints or 2 pounds daily (dependent on fluid intake). It eliminates some fluid which is converted into urine. It is affected in diabetes as unprocessed sugar is passed into the urine. It can be the seat of kidney stones (calcium salts and uric acid, crystallized), infections (since the nephrons or filters become prone to the substances filtered). It affects and is affected by high and low blood pressure (the more blood enters the kidney the more overworked it is - the more fluid is left behind in the tissues, which is then called edema, the less blood pumped to the kidney the less efficient it is at draining fluid from tissues, resulting in edema from low blood pressure), gout, (uric acid is not properly removed from the blood and settles in a joint, often in the big toe), arthritis (again, improper filtering of acids detrimental to the joints), eye problems (improper correlation of liver

At the waist, between the 2nd and 3rd toes, about one thumb-width above the waist and one thumb-width below it, will adequately encompass the kidney reflex, which is lower in the right foot (pressed down by the liver) and longer in males. Use your thumb to work the reflex in *kidney* shape, "(" on the right foot, ")," on the left foot. Or you can locate the reflex differently; run your index finger down the foot from the solar plexus reflex to the heel, swiftly and firmly down the centre of the foot. You will encounter a lump or harder or fleshier mound, often near the waist of the foot. This *lump* is the kidney reflex. This method is used to locate a *floating* kidney.

For kidney stones, work the entire foot, then the urinary system, exclusively, backwards and forwards, from bladder to ureter tube to kidney, and back again, for at least an hour. Have your client go home to take a long warm bath, making sure that no stress is allowed to affect her at all. Have her drink lots of water. Have a companion massage her hands, arms, legs and back repeatedly for relaxation;

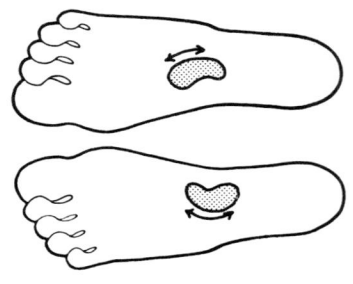

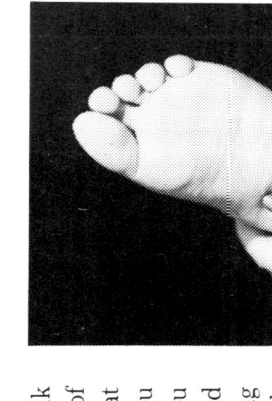

(Kidney, cont.)

and kidney to drain lactic acid).
-Vitamin A,B6 and C, all Minerals especially Potassium and Calcium, Lemon Juice, Water, Parsley, Horsetail and Cornsilk Teas, Watermelon Seeds ground and used as tea, Cranberry Juice. Limit cooked Spinach, Rhubarb and Cranberries when there is a kidney problem as they are high in oxalic acid. Limit coffee, sweet juices and fruit.

especially when she is in her warm bath. The companion must screen her from children, stressful phone calls etc. She must be totally relaxed. Repeat the Reflexology session on the following day, and the next, until the stone leaves the kidney and ureter tube to enter the bladder, where it will be passed easily. The foot will be extremely sensitive, work gently and caringly, but keep working the same reflexes until the stone leaves. This set of reflexes has been extremely effective for the total relaxation of the client, allowing a relaxed passageway for the stone to leave.

Ureter Tubes
-lower abdominal cavity, pelvic area
-both feet
-*urinary system*

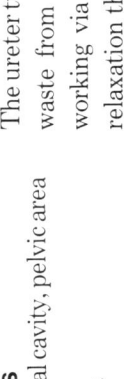

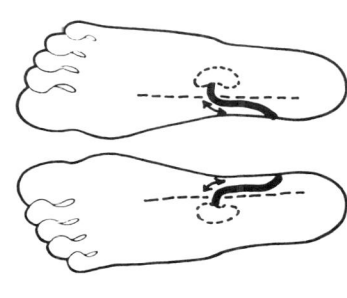

The ureter tubes are a channel that carry waste from the kidney to the bladder, working via muscular contractions and relaxation that squeeze the urine down.

From the kidney reflex at the waist, walk your thumb toward the medial side of the foot, until it crosses the tendon that extends from the big toe downward. You can feel and expose the tendon when you push the client's big toe toward him, and must avoid working on it. Lounge along the tendon on its medial side, to the heel. You may walk alongside the tendon in either direction from waist to heel or heel to waist.

MOSTLY THE SIDES OF THE FOOT

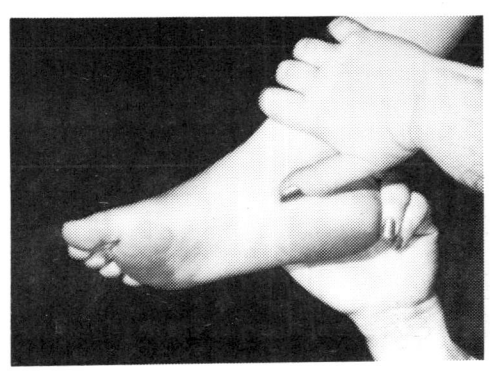

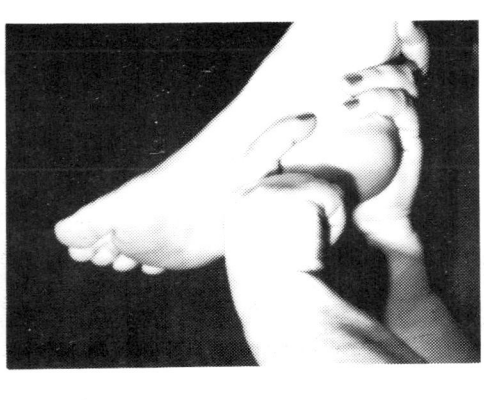

(see pictures below)

Bladder
-pelvic area
-both feet
-urinary system

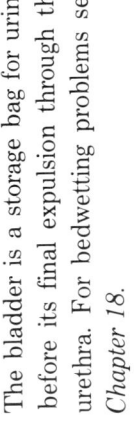

The bladder is a storage bag for urine before its final expulsion through the urethra. For bedwetting problems see *Chapter 18.*

Look for a puffy area on the medial side of the foot, near the heel, on the *side* of the foot, not the plantar surface.

In some people it may appear swollen, puffy and red, denoting possible bladder problems. Work the entire puffy area from all directions with thumbs or fingers. Generally, you will find it easier to work the urinary system from bladder to ureter tube to kidney, but it makes no real difference.

Urethra, Penis, Vagina
-pelvic area
-both feet
-urinary system

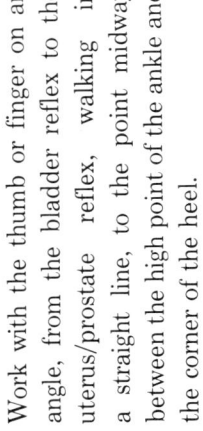

The urethra carries urine out of the body, and, in the male, allows semen to flow out of the body.

Work with the thumb or finger on an angle, from the bladder reflex to the uterus/prostate reflex, walking in a straight line, to the point midway between the high point of the ankle and the corner of the heel.

NOTE: The reflex to the *prostate/uterus* is explained on pages 72 and 73 and can be done either at this point, or in the sequence given.

Inguinal Lymph Nodes
-pelvic area in groin
-both feet
-lymphatic system

The lymph nodes in the groin protect the body, the abdominal area and the pelvic area from toxins, disseminate antibodies where needed, and aid the circulatory system to feed cells and remove wastes through its own lymphatic vessels.

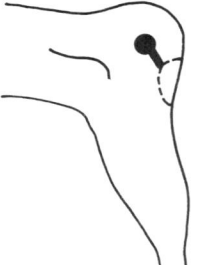

Your thumbs will press on the ball of the foot, to push your client's foot toward her, allowing the tendons in the ankle to stand out. If your client is flexing her own foot, this *WILL NOT WORK.* Your fingers will not be able to pass through

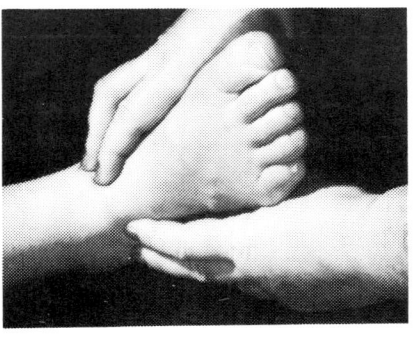
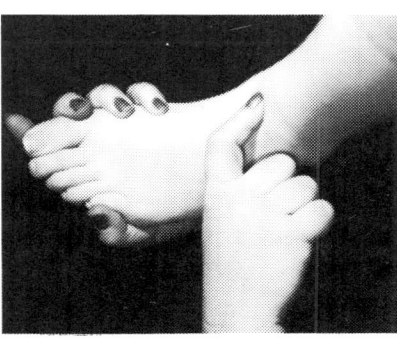
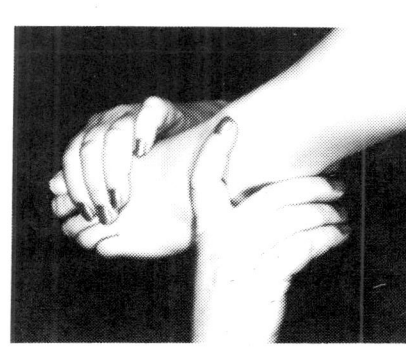

(Inguinal Lymph, cont.)

There are twice as many lymph vessels in the body as blood vessels. The nodes filter wastes, holding them until they can be eliminated through eliminative organs; lung, skin, kidney and bowel. The groin lymphatics drain fluid from the legs, feet and pelvic area. Lymph itself is a colourless fluid that drains into the brachio-cephalic vein at the side of the neck. Three quarters of the body drains its lymph on the left side, one quarter is drained on the right side (drain plug).

Lymph flows because of body motion and exercise. It has no pump as does the blood. Lymph vessels flow near veins to aid the cirulatory system. Lymph left undrained can cause swelling in the tissues, lumpy areas under the skin. Massage of these lumps can return the flow of lymph, dispersing the puffiness, as can dry brush massage.

-Vitamin A,B6 and C, Lecithin, Cider Vinegar, Fenugreek, Cayenne, Red Sage, Parsley, Chapparral, Dandelion.

the muscle band in the ankle. She must be passive. The indexes of both your hands will walk between the tendons in the ankle area from the base of the ankle bone to the top of the ankle bone, a distance of 1 to 2 inches, in between all the tendons of the ankle area, walking upwards. The lymph in the groin or the inguinal node reflex is always worked upwards, toward the heart.

Now, one index will hook in at the centre of the ankle, in the inguinal region, and you will alternately flex the foot, hooking in deep, and extend the foot, releasing pressure. This is called the *Lymph Push/ Pull.* Note that you must always follow work on the lymph in the groin with the *drain plug* reflex and lymph drainage from the knee.

Start at the knee, with the index finger tracing a line along the *inside* of the leg, at the bone's lower edge, aimed into the bone. Continue to trace the line over the ankle, over the top of the foot, heading straight for the inner corner of the big toe, where you will hook in with the index finger, on the dorsal side of the toe, thumb on the plantar side of the toe for the *drain plug.* Hook in only once on each surface, up and into the bone of the big toe. (See *Drain Plug, Lymphatic Drainage* page 37.) Remember the lymph nodes to head and neck and axillary lymphatics at armpit.

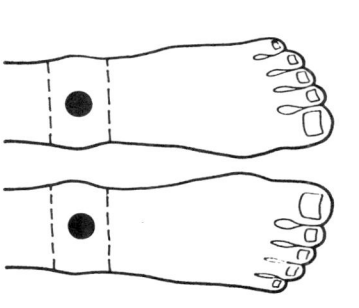

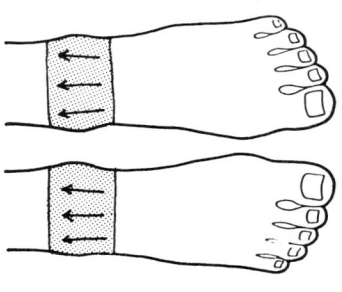

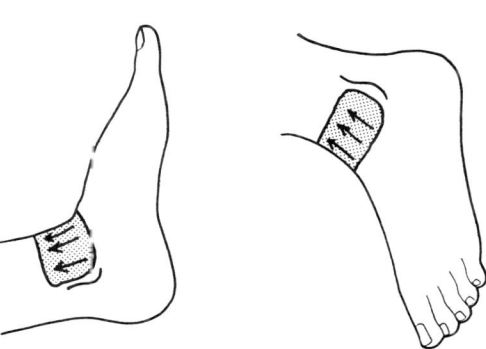

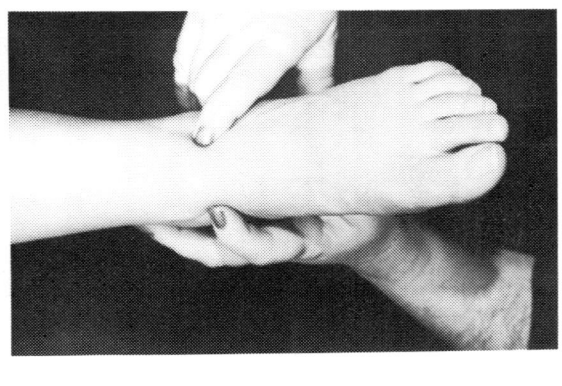
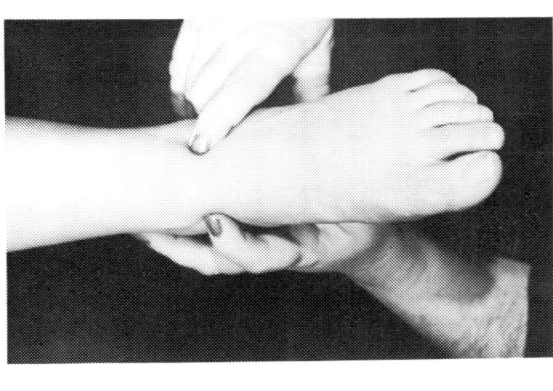

Lymphatic Pull

The *lymphatic pull* is the next stage of working the lymphatic reflexes, even though it is on the plantar surface. Stretch the muscles below the skin, from the heel to the top of the ball of the foot, near the lateral edge of the foot, below the 5th toe in the 5th zone. First take small bites to stretch the skin adding in small areas until you are streching the entire area from heel to shoulder joint reflex. Then, repeat the same motion, but from the shoulder joint reflex across the top of the ball of the foot to the big toe. Give a good final stretch to each *pull.*

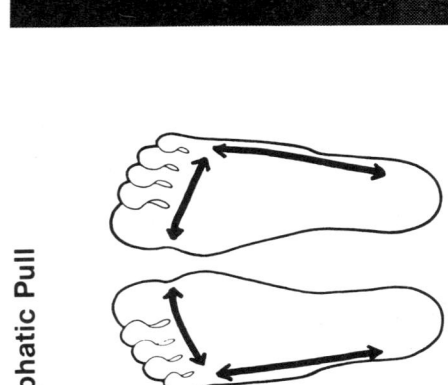
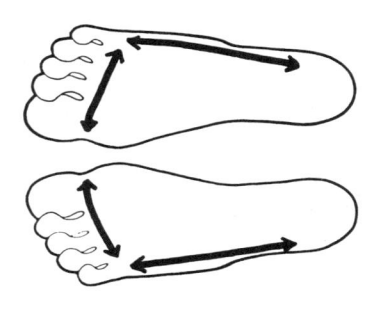
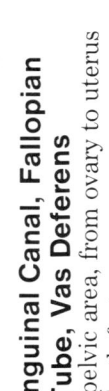
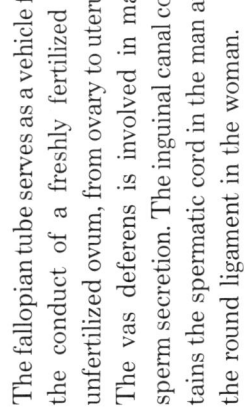

Inguinal Canal, Fallopian Tube, Vas Deferens
-pelvic area, from ovary to uterus
-both feet
-reproductive system

The fallopian tube serves as a vehicle for the conduct of a freshly fertilized or unfertilized ovum, from ovary to uterus. The vas deferens is involved in male sperm secretion. The inguinal canal contains the spermatic cord in the man and the round ligament in the woman.

For either reflex, walk your thumb in either direction from the base of the ankle bone on one side to the ankle bone's base on the other side, right where the foot bends, at the base of the reflex to the inguinal nodes. Note any puffiness that is encountered, which might denote edema or problems in the reproductive tract. Gently press any fluid up the leg towards the heart.

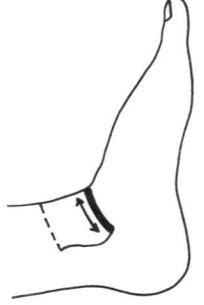
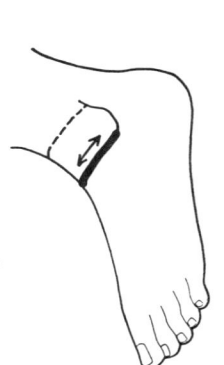
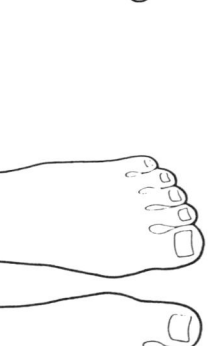
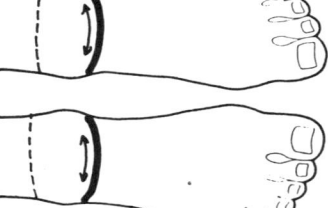

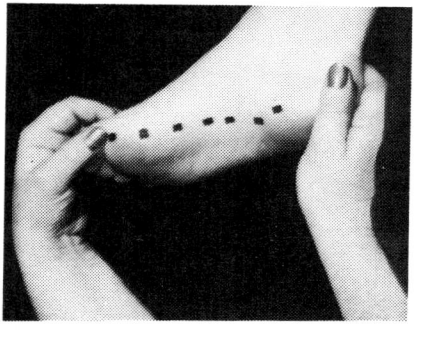
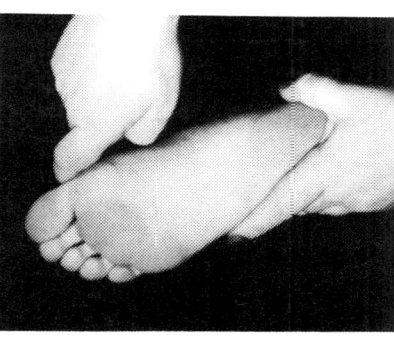
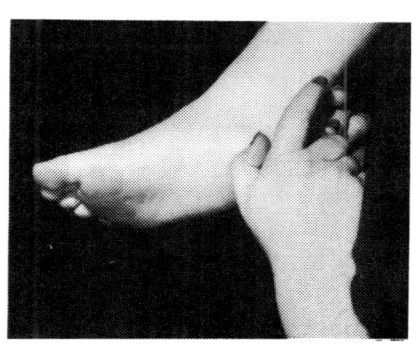

Spine

-centre of back, attaching skull, ribs, pelvic girdle
-7 cervicals, 12 thoracic, 5 lumbar, 1 sacrum, 1 coccyx
-both feet
-*nervous and structural system*

The spine is a collection of 26 articulated bones, separated by spongy discs, held together and kept upright by muscles and ligaments. It is the housing for the spinal cord, which conveys millions of bits of information to and from the body and brain, for motion, response, and function of all parts of the system. Four curves in the spine allow movement and eliminate shock of movement, distributing the weight of torso and head. Arising from the spinal cord are spinal nerves, emerging through openings between the vertebrae. In the chest area each pair of spinal nerves is specialized for specific parts and organs. Elsewhere, nerves subdivide to form networks (plexii). The autonomic nervous system activates involuntary smooth and cardiac muscles and glands serving vital organ systems, digestive, cirulatory, respiratory, urinary, reproductive and endocrine. The autonomic nervous system is divided into sympathetic and parasympathetic systems, which oppose each other in function to balance the body's activities. Parasympathetic fibers to the heart, slow down the heart beat, sympathetic fibers to the heart accelerate it; the former constrict the bronchii, the latter dilate them.

These divisions together regulate bladder response, respiratory and heart rate, blood flow and pressure, temperature, digestive, liver and intestinal functions and endocrine glands. For the proper function of the nervous system, you need a proper spine and therefore,

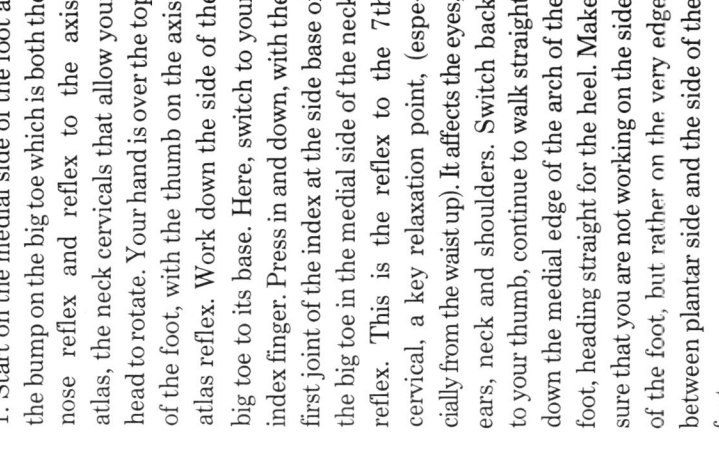

There are three ways to work the spinal reflexes. Work all of them.

1. Start on the medial side of the foot at the bump on the big toe which is both the nose reflex and reflex to the axis-atlas, the neck cervicals that allow your head to rotate. Your hand is over the top of the foot, with the thumb on the axis-atlas reflex. Work down the side of the big toe to its base. Here, switch to your index finger. Press in and down, with the first joint of the index at the side base of the big toe in the medial side of the neck reflex. This is the reflex to the 7th cervical, a key relaxation point, (especially from the waist up). It affects the eyes, ears, neck and shoulders. Switch back to your thumb, continue to walk straight down the medial edge of the arch of the foot, heading straight for the heel. Make sure that you are not working on the side of the foot, but rather on the very edge between plantar side and the side of the foot.

Switch to your other thumb and hook in with the entire side of your thumb so that the outside of it is lying along the *SIDE* edge of the heel (*not* the plantar surface). This is the coccyx reflex, another key relaxation point, from the waist down, affecting the reproductive system, bowels, and strangely enough, the eyes, ears, nose and throat. The coccyx and 7th cervical affect the energy that moves up the spine. Holding both simultaneously, very lightly, revives and renews the energy cycles in the body. (see Desserts, Chapter 12.) Wait for an even

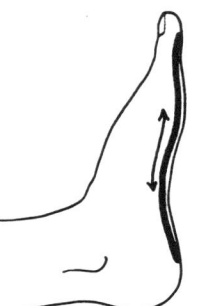
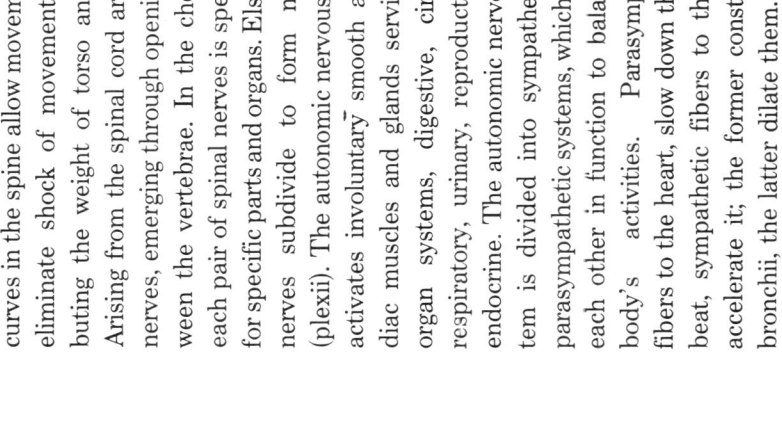

(continued over)

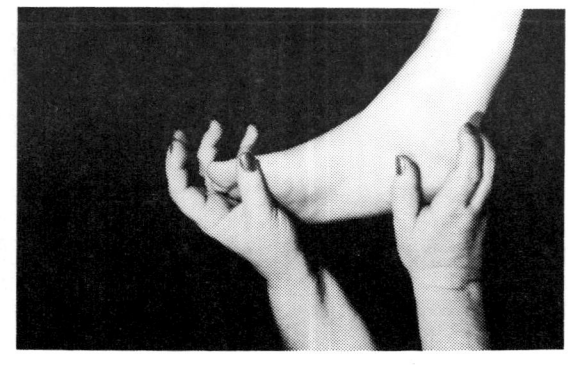

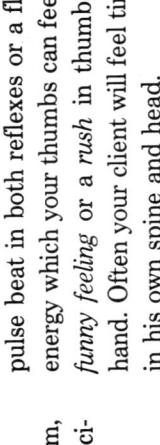

(Spine, cont.)

proper musculature.
-All Vitamins, Calcium, Magnesium, Manganese, Iron, Zinc, Copper, Lecithin, Cayenne.

pulse beat in both reflexes or a flow of energy which your thumbs can feel as a *funny feeling* or a *rush* in thumbs and hand. Often your client will feel tingling in his own spine and head.

2. Your hand is anchored on the top of the foot, your thumb on the axis/atlas reflex as before and you walk down cervicals and 7th cervical. But now, note the bony structure on the medial side of the foot, from the *bunion* area or top of first metatarsal bone, to the ankle bone. Your thumb will hook in, below the bone and at a 45 degree angle into it as it comes from above the bone, and hooks up under it along its length to the ankle bone, around the base of the ankle, and then up the side of the leg, for about 6 inches. From axis/atlas reflex to the 7th cervical reflex are the reflexes to the 7 cervicals. From the 7th cervical reflex to the bony protrusion on the side of the foot, along the bone line (Cuneiform I) represents the thoracic vertebrae. The soft, boneless area between protrusion and ankle bone is the lumbar reflex. The sacrum reflex is at the base of the ankle followed by the reflex to the coccyx, around the ankle. You may work this reflex from coccyx to axis/atlas, back and forth. It is generally very sensitive so work with concern for your client.

Reflexes 1 and 2 can both be worked from either direction. If you curve away from the sacrum coccyx reflex to come up around the forward part of the ankle bone, you are working the symphysis pubis, the front portion of the pelvic bones.

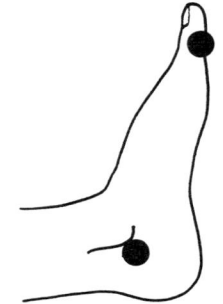

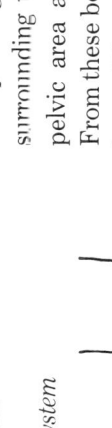

(Spine, cont.)

3. In this spinal reflex, your thumb will come in perpendicular to the two previous reflexes, and walk across both of them. In other words you are walking your thumb from dorsal to plantar surface, crossing both spinal reflexes, starting below the big toe and ending at the line from ankle to heel. You may work from top to bottom of foot or bottom to top, with either thumb. This is the most gentle and comfortable of the spinal reflexes.

If you encounter a sore spot in the spinal reflex, you can lay the spinal reflex of *YOUR* thumb along the sensitive area and it will remove much of the sensitivity. Or, on the medial side, brush the skin gently from ankle to toe. On the lateral side brush upward from little toe past ankle. This is a pain removal technique which affects the acupuncture meridians and reduces pain.

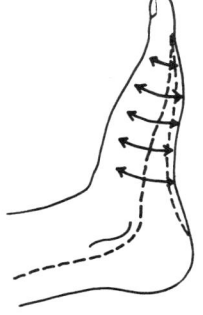

Pelvic Girdle
-pelvic area
-structural system

The pelvic girdle is a bony structure surrounding the internal organs in the pelvic area and supporting the spine. From these bones are attached the thigh bones. The pelvic girdle and the sacrum together give man the ability to walk erect.

The pelvic girdle reflex is a large one that starts at the inner corner of the ankle bone, medial side, surrounds the base of it, then goes midway between ankle bone and heel, embracing urethra, prostate/ uterus reflexes flowing in a gentle curve that simulates the curve of the heel, but doesn't reach to it. The entire area is gently worked with the thumb or fingers. The same reflex, in the same shape, will be found on the lateral side of the foot and is worked the same way.

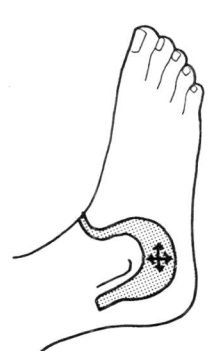

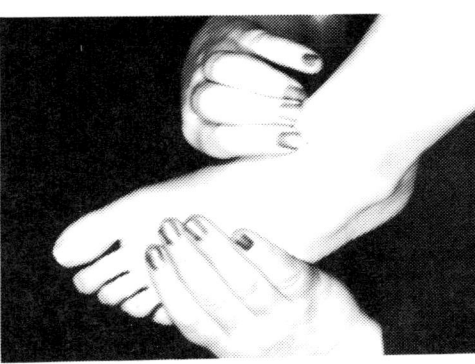

(see picture below)

Pubic Symphesis
-pelvic area
-both feet
-structural system

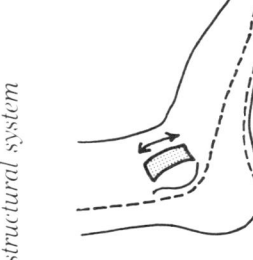

The joining of the pelvic bone in the front of the body at the base of the pelvis forms a strong supportive arch.

With your thumb, work along the front of the medial ankle bone in an upward curve for the pubic symphesis.

Ovaries/Uterus
(female reproductive organs)
-pelvic area
-both feet
-endocrine system

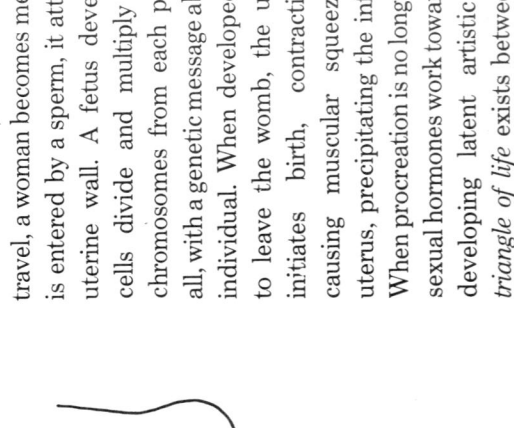

The ovaries and uterus are procreative and creative glands, as well as are the testes and prostate. The ovaries produce the eggs which leave one at a time, monthly, from the ovary, to enter the fallopian tube upon command from the pituitary gland. If it is unfertilized and does not attach to the uterine wall in its travel, a woman becomes menstrual. If it is entered by a sperm, it attaches to the uterine wall. A fetus develops as the cells divide and multiply sharing 23 chromosomes from each parent, 46 in all, with a genetic message about the new individual. When developed and ready to leave the womb, the unborn child initiates birth, contractions occur, causing muscular squeezing of the uterus, precipitating the infant's birth. When procreation is no longer a concern, sexual hormones work toward creativity, developing latent artistic talents. A *triangle of life* exists between the pitui-

The reflex to the uterus and prostate are the same. Place your ring finger on the very corner of the heel. Now line up your middle finger to form a straight line with the other two fingers and equi-distant from them. Place the thumb of the same hand on the spot occupied by the middle finger, and remove all fingers but the thumb. Cup the heel with the fingers just removed as you hook in very gently with your thumb. This is the best (to date) measuring method to locate the sex glands.

The uterus/prostate reflex is the centre point between the high point of the heel and the corner of the heel if a straight line were drawn through the three points.

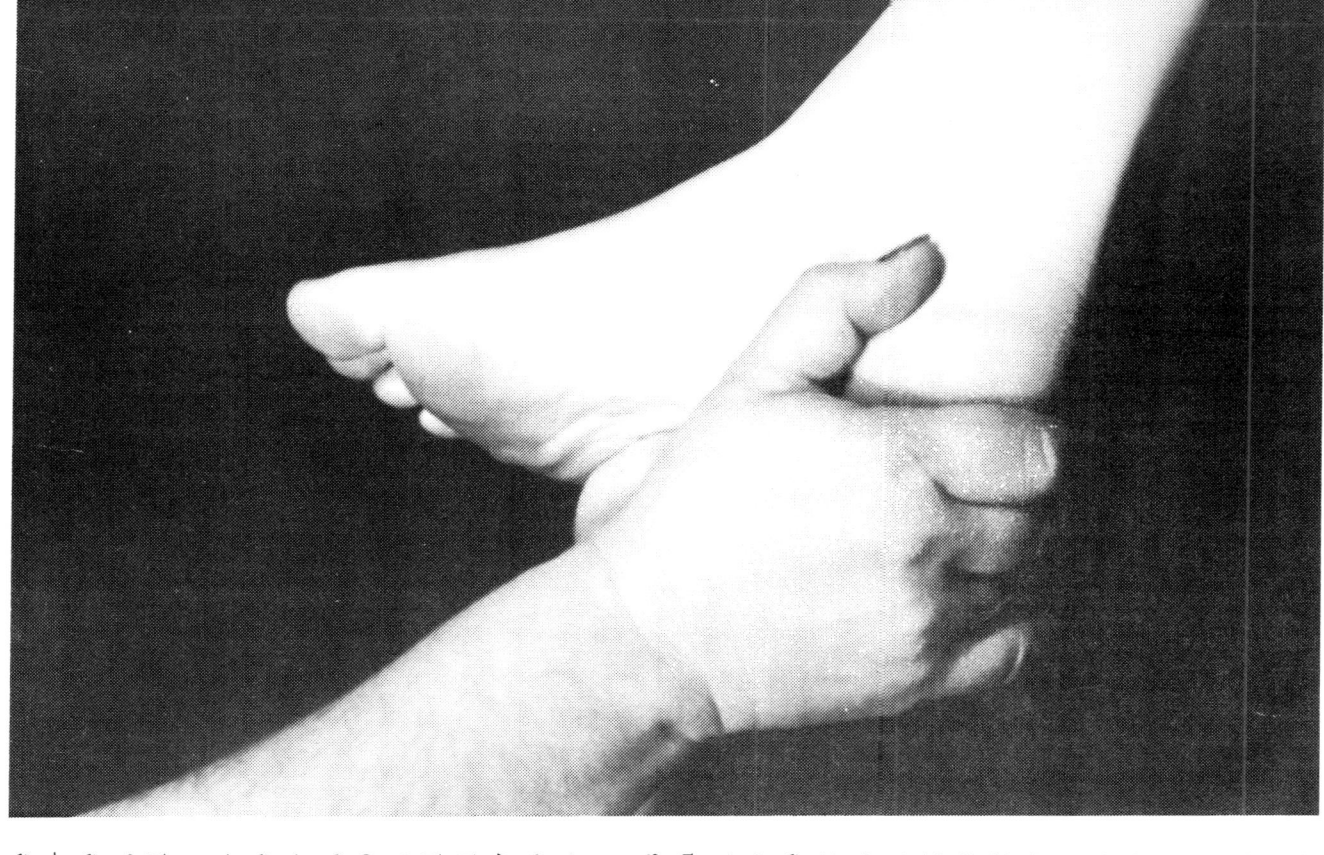

tary gland and the gonads. With the removal of any sexual organ, the pituitary gland becomes shaky, until the thyroid and adrenal glands support it, and may be the cause of emotional distress after surgery.

This *triangle* affects growth, moods, sexuality, childbearing, emotions, voice tone, skin, and general health. Testosterone is produced by the adrenal glands, inhibited by the ovaries and turned into estrogen (female hormone) when needed. Follicles in the ovaries produce estradiol and other estrogens, involved in cell respiration, blood circulation, and primary and secondary sex characteristics. The corpus luteum manufactures progesterone.

Testes/Prostate (male reproductive organs)
-pelvic area
-both feet
-*endocrine system*

The male reproductive system consists of the testes (suspended in a sack of skin called the scrotum), a series of ducts and a number of glands. Development of the male germinating cells, sperm, in the testes, requires a temperature of about 35 degrees celsius. The scrotum stores them at this temperature, extending and drawing in toward the body, depending on surrounding heat or cold. Sperm cells move through the vas deferens, passing through the abdominal wall and pelvic cavity to enter the prostatic urethra. Here the nutrient-rich secretions of the prostate gland and seminal vessicles are added to the sperm to form semen.

The testes are glands that arise on the posterior abdominal wall during fetal development. As the body lengthens, these organs seem to descend. Actually

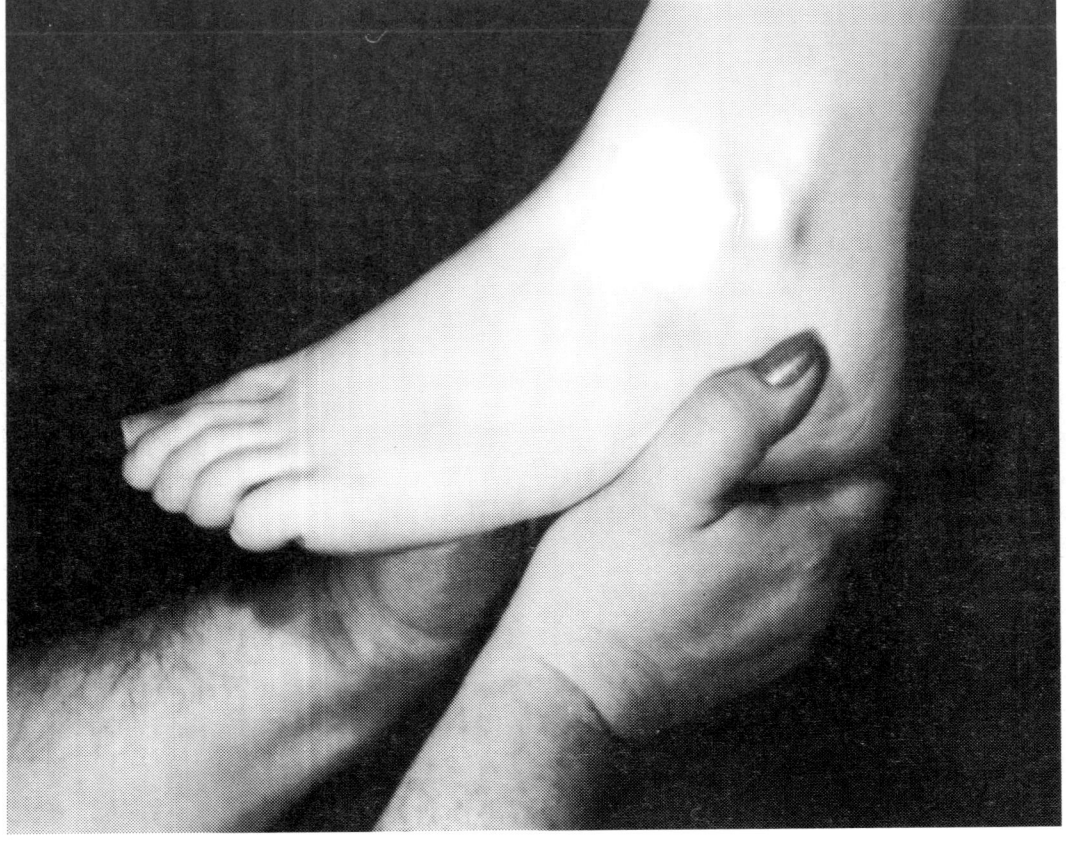

The reflex to the ovary/testes is the same. They are located on the lateral side of the foot. Using index, middle and ring fingers in a straight line, replace middle finger with your thumb and cup the heel with your hand as you hook in

(Testes/Prostate cont.)

they don't. The testes have two functions - the development and excretion of sperm and the secretion of testosterone, the male sex hormone (also produced in women and valuable for muscular strength).

A mature sperm cell contains 23 chromosomes in its nucleus, enzymes to break down barriers around the ovum, mitochondria to power the cell, and a tail to propel it. Testosterone stimulates the ducts and glands at puberty as well as body hair, voice tone and larynx structure and is influenced by the pituitary gland. The prostate gland whose alkaline secretions activate the sperm, can become inflamed and painful, causing difficult urination.

The urethra in the male has 3 parts. The prostatic portion receives urine from the urinary bladder, sperm from the ejaculatory ducts, and secretions from the prostate via several ducts. A neuromuscular mechanism prevents voiding of urine during the production of semen. The urethra has mucous secreting glands.

Although the ovaries and testes share a common origin, as do the male and female external genital features, the uterus, its tubes and the upper two-thirds of the vagina rise from a duct system different from that in the male. When there is trouble in the sex glands, check the neck. Often fusion of the vertebrae in the neck will affect uterus or prostate. Also check for prolapsed colon

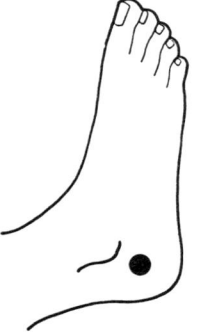

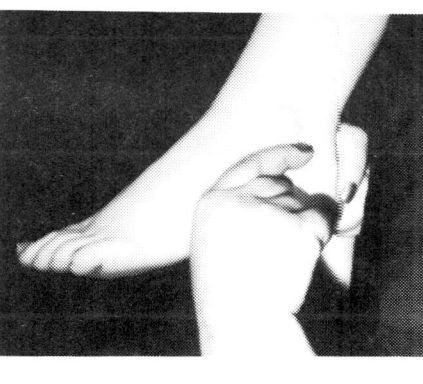 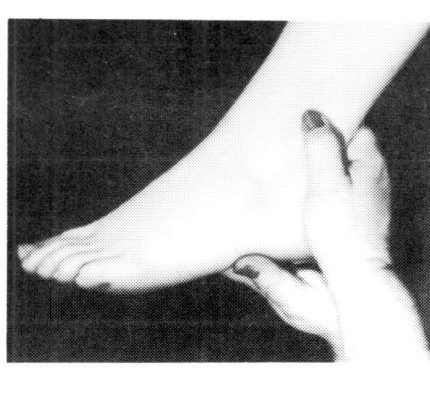

gently.

In the woman, the reflexes to the ovaries and uterus are generally sensitive on one or both feet, since the woman is always in a state of flux, with ovulation, menstruation, menopause, etc...

If the reflex is sensitive in the man, ask whether he uses a zinc supplement and suggest that some people have healed their prostate gland with its use or with a daily handful of pumpkin seeds.

or low back problems in lumbar and sacral regions.

-All Vitamins, especially E, B6 and A, Nucleoproteins, Minerals, specifically Zinc (Pumpkin Seeds, Sunflower Seeds, Oysters).

Female: Black Cohosh, Raspberry, Licorish, Dang Quei.

Male: Ginseng, Juniper Berry, Golden Seal, Marshmallow.

Sex Drive: Damiana, Ginseng.

There are two reflexes to the hip as well as a referred area, which is the shoulder joint itself.

1. On the lateral side of the foot, just below the ankle bone. Use your index finger to hook in and walk under the ankle bone, hooking it at a 45 degree angle from the front of the ankle bone to the back of it. You can also work from the back to the front of the ankle bone by coming in from behind the heel with your index finger of the other hand while cupping the heel with the fingers of that hand. You can also work up the outside of the leg about six inches between the side of the achilles heel and the calf muscles.

This is also a reflex to the low back and the sciatic nerve.

2. Look at the lateral side of the foot. Note the bone that delineates the waist and the bone that is within the heel (talus). Below and in front of the lateral ankle bone bounded by the two bones mentioned is a *soft triangle* that is not bony. Work this whole triangle with any

The hip often affects and is affected by shoulder problems, sciatic problems, knee problems and things as distant as jaw problems.

-Vitamin A, D and E, Calcium, Magnesium, Manganese, Lecithin.

Hip

-pelvic area, attached to sacrum
-both feet
-*structural system*

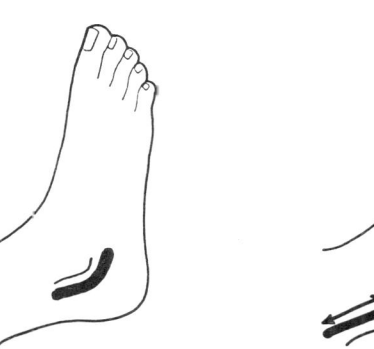 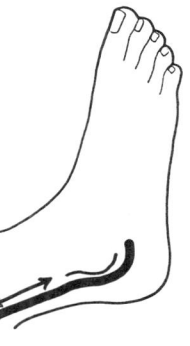

(continued on next page)

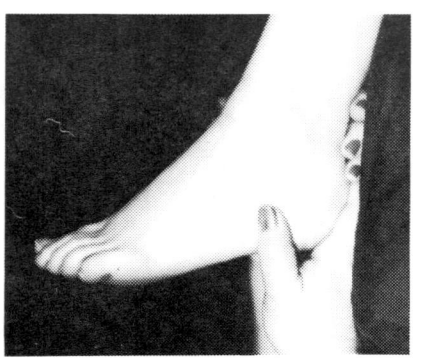
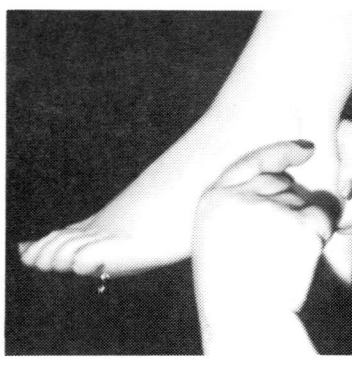
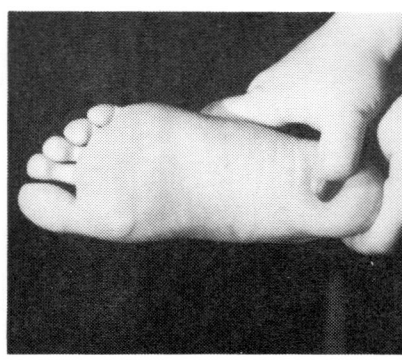

(Hip cont.)

available finger in all directions. This is also a reflex to the low back, the knee and the elbow.

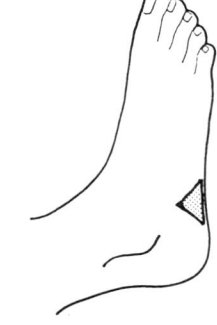
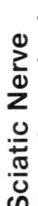

Sciatic Nerve

-from lower lumbar or sacrum, down back of buttock and leg to foot
-both feet
-nervous system

The sciatic nerve is the largest nerve in the body, existing at the lumbar sacral area, dividing several times, supplying muscular nerves as it passes down the leg to straddle the heel. It affects and is affected by the hip, shoulder, neck problems, or jaw joint displacement (TMJ). -Vitamin B Complex and E, Calcium, Magnesium, Manganese.

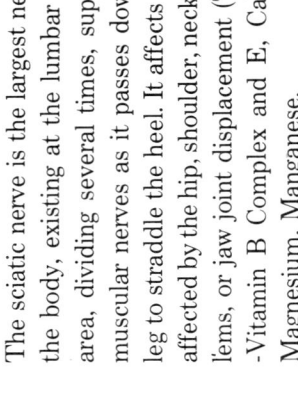

The reflex to the sciatic nerve is the same as reflex 1 to the hip. Use your index finger at a 45 degree angle into the base of the outer ankle bone, from front to back or back to front. Then go up the side of the leg about 6 inches.

2. The reflex to the sciatic that is just below the very centre of the heel is difficult to reach because of the thickness of the skin on the heel and its callouses.

3. Below the ankle bone, slightly lower and in front of ovary/testes reflex.

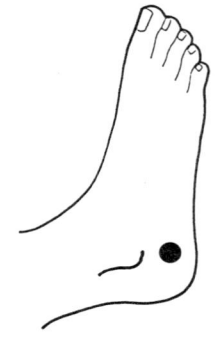

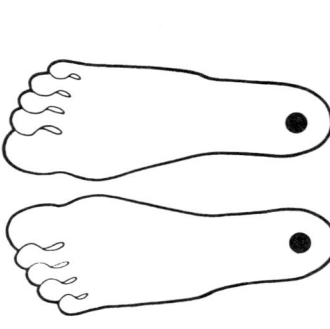
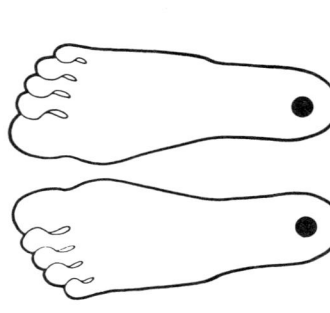

Knee
-between thigh and leg
-both feet
-*structural system*

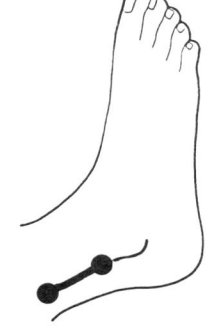

The knee often affects and is affected by the hip, foot and leg problems. Jogging, heavy sports, kneeling, and sports such as tennis or raquetball often jar the knee excessively, especially if no stretching or warm-up exercises are done first.
-Vitamin A, D and E, Calcium, Magnesium, Manganese, Lecithin.

The knee reflex is in the *soft triangle* along with the hip and low back reflex. It is also represented by the bone on the lateral side of the foot that denotes the waist of the foot. You can also work the referred reflex in the elbow remembering that they bend differently, so if there is pain on the big toe side of the knee, work the thumb side of elbow, back part of knee equals the soft inside of elbow. Pinky toe = pinky finger side.

Elbow
-arm joint
-both feet
-*structural system*

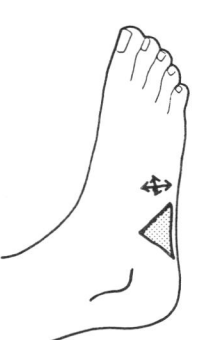

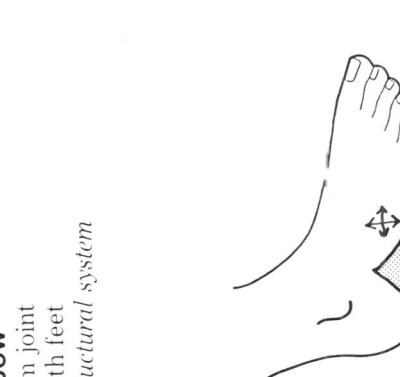

The elbow takes a great beating in all sports and general work and is affected by hand, arm, shoulder, neck and chest muscles.
For all joints use All Vitamins, Minerals, especially Vitamin A and D, Calcium, Lecithin and Comfrey.

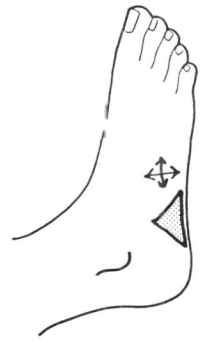

The elbow reflex is the same as the knee reflex in the *soft triangle* below the ankle, at the *waistbone* of the foot, and as a referred reflex work the knee, or the opposite elbow.

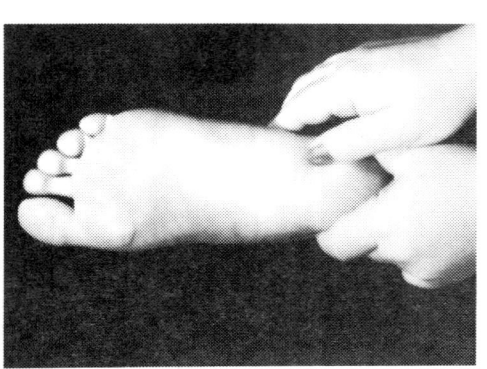

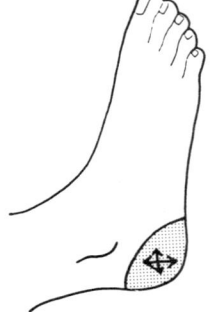

Work the thumbs in a semi-circle at the heel edge of the lateral side of the foot around its corner, taking in the reflexes to the testes and ovaries.

(see picture below)

Arm/Leg
-extremities
-both feet
-*structural system*

Used to walk in conjunction with each other for balanced walking and in the performance of all activities.

Arms may be affected by the shoulder, neck, back of chest muscles; the legs may be affected by hip, buttocks, low back, and foot muscles.

Buttock
-pelvic, behind hip
-both feet
-*structural system*

Gluteus medius and gluteus maximus muscles affect walking, sitting, the legs, the torso and most movement.

Foot
-end of leg, extremities
-both feet
-*structural system*

The foot is the foundation of your body. If it suffers or weakens, the pain or dis-equilibrium may reflect to other parts of the body. If the arch drops or is too high, check for back problems. If the big toe is too stiff, calloused or painful, refer to the neck. If the heel is calloused, check for hip discomfort. If there is redness or

For the actual foot reflex, press deeply into the centre line of the lower portion of the heel. Also work the lateral zone reflex on the opposite foot.

Work individual fingers for the toes or their lateral counterpart.

Work the palm for the foot's plantar surface and the back of the hand for the

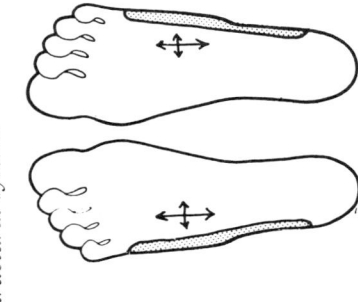

78

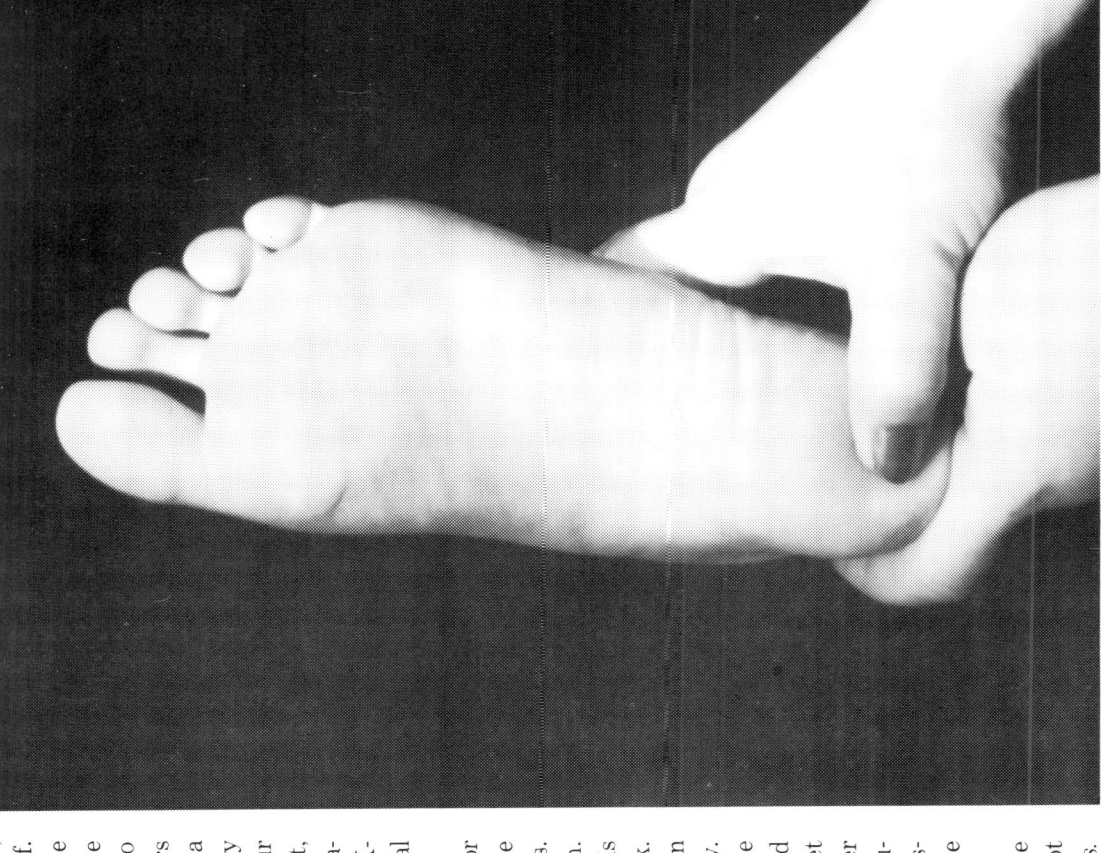

dorsum of the foot.
For ankle problems, work on the wrist. For the gaits press in deeply at the points pictured on both feet or as shown on page 124.

puffiness on the bladder reflex, check for bladder infection. Does the foot look squeezed into shoes? The person's gait may be *off*. Stretch it outward and upward to unsqueeze it. Callouses may indicate uneven leg length, tilted pelvis, and the body's attempt to equalize itself. Look closely at the foot, it contains the key to the body as well as being the medium from which you work. Be kind to the foot, no one else is! Save powders and lotions and bathing for after a session, since they cut off the energy flow, cause fingers to slip, and fool your sense of the foot's state of tension, heat, and skin tone. Refer people to a podiatrist for podiatric problems and to an X-ray lab if you suspect a break or internal injury.

The body depends on proper care for each area; check people's shoes and the tightness of their socks and stockings. That alone might solve a back problem. A *Health Shoe* is one that fits; all else is someone's money making gimmick. Walking barefoot on sand and uneven ground is the best form of Reflexology. Hot and cold alternating baths help the foot in pain and are an aid to sleep, and improve circulation. Pained feet improve in a bath of potato-skin water (potassium broth). Leg muscles influence the foot, so extend your compression technique up the leg, right to the knee, on all parts of the leg.
Work the hand for foot problems and the foot for hand problems. Is the foot odorous? Check the liver and think *stress*.

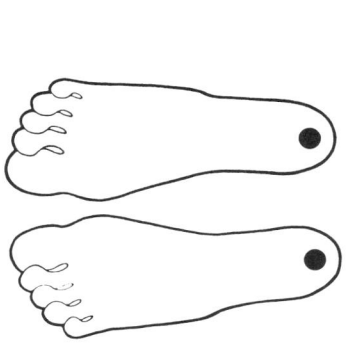
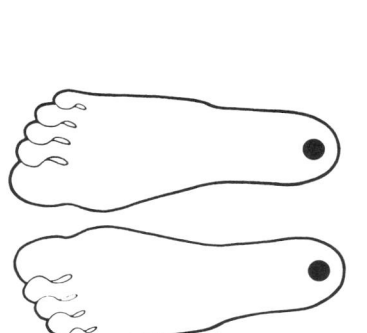
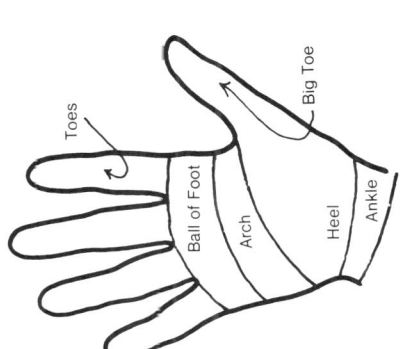

(continued on next page)

79

(Foot, cont.)

Puffy ankles? Check the lymphatics and kidney, be aware of possible blood pressure problems and brush and caress the tissue fluid upward toward the heart.

Hand
-end of arm, extremity
-both feet
-*structural system*

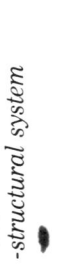

Where the foot is structured to support the body's weight and to provide a mobile platform for many activities on many terrains, the hand with its long fingers, slightly lighter bones and great flexibility, is more of a tool or machine for more precise functions, with incredible dexterity. Its use and flexibility provide many clues to a person's health condition and nature. Tremors may indicate thyroid malfunction, adrenal exhaustion, as may skin tone and texture. Nails may speak of the body's mineral content; white spots on nails may indicate lack of zinc, calcium deficiency or undue stress. Thumb rigidity may indicate a person's rigidity, poor acceptance of new ideas, trust as well as head and neck problems. A *dead* hand may mean energy drain and possible *overcharge* in a major system.

To work on the hand, work on the referred reflex in the foot, or on the other hand, (lateral reflex). For the fingers, work on the toes or on the opposite fingers. If the wrist hurts, work on the ankle or on the opposite wrist. Never work on the injured hand itself as it may compound the problem.

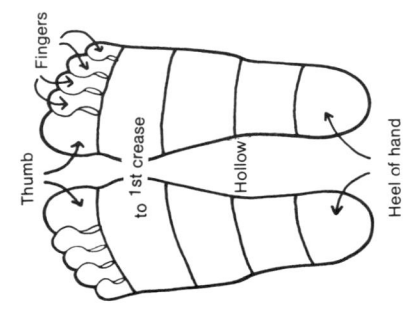

The following explanations are not palmistry, but are pure common sense and observation.

Flexibility	The hand should be flexible, but not limp; movable, but with a bit of resistance, especially if you are touching the hand for the first time. Too much trust in anyone is as ineffective as no trust at all. Limpness may indicate a weak constitution, lack of desires, energy loss.
Resilience	A hand with no *body* may indicate poor resistance to disease and to life's ups and downs.
Thumb rigid	Lack of trust, inability to change, stiff neckedness, neck or back problems.
Thumb lax	Abdication of responsibility (even for his own health), person needs mothering, diseases corresponding to *good mothering* might be prevalent.

COLOUR

very red	Circulatory problems (heat, blood).
very white	Lymph and nerve problems.

LINES

Red Gashes	Over-energized person, over-emotional. This person may need help to become aware of his limitations so that he can allow his body to catch up. He may also have unnoticed pain, therefore over-taxes himself.
Faint	(In a sturdy hand) Repressed person, constipation, blow-ups and breakdowns.
Strong	(In a small hand) High energy, taking its toll on the body.

NAILS

Shattered	Energy is scattered.
Bluish	Poor circulation.
Split	Arthritis, rheumatism, teeth, bowel trouble, energy dissipation.
Brittle (no moons)	Underactive thyroid.
Long, shiny, narrow (large moons)	Overactive thyroid.
White spots	Zinc or calcium deficiency, and/or undue stress, too much sugar consumed.
Lumpy	Foreign bodies in system, cellulite, *lumpy* muscles.
Vertical lines	Unhealthy fiber.
Horizontal lines	Blockages of energy, acute illness.
Wavy lines	Older dis-ease.
Thin	Sensitivity.
Short, flat	High blood pressure, aggressiveness.
Spoon	Glandular disorder.
White	(When hand is stretched) Anaemia.
Rough	Drug use, sexual problems, confused thought processes.

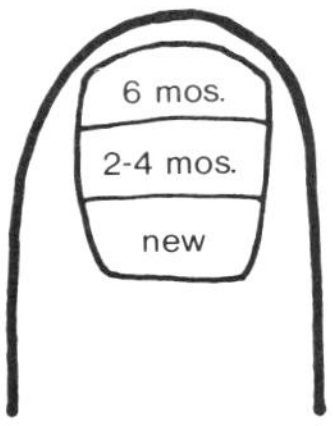

Nails take six months to grow out. An adequate time sequence may be observed by noting where in the nail the problem occurs.

FINGERS

Big knuckles	(Not always apparent, feel for them.) Anxiety, nervous disorder, constipation, slow reactions, arthritic possibility, filtering of incoming and outgoing information.
Small knuckles	Hysterical reactions, over-reaction in situations, involvement in strange situations before being aware of them.
Short index	Ulcers, hypertension.
Enlarged lower phalange	Gout, rheumatism.
Crooked ring finger	Heart problems, sexual problems.
Swollen fingers	High blood pressure.

(nail diagram labels: 6 mos. / 2-4 mos. / new)

Tips of fingers
Lower phallanges
Fingers red, purple,
painful, nails chipped,
broken, weak
Man's hand swollen

Top of the body – brain.
Sexual organs.

Poor thinking, poor generation of sexual energy.
Too much drinking, kidney, heart swollen.
If you cannot make an indentation between the knuckles when your hand makes a fist, there might be hardening of the arteries and/or a problem with the kidneys.

Look carefully at the hands, make comparisons and learn your own identification points. All of the specifications made here are flexible. If you are discerning you will be able to compare them with what you've already learned from observation and work on feet. Remember *NOT TO DIAGNOSE.* The points mentioned are for your information and your direction.

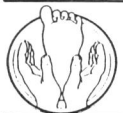

Chapter 14
QUESTIONS ON ARCHITECTURE OF THE FOOT

Which gland is both an endocrine and an exocrine gland? _____

There is a *Master Gland* and an organ called *King of the Glands*. The Master Gland is _____ the King of the Glands is _____.

The tonsils protect the spine and the bronchials. TRUE_____FALSE_____

Mark the 5 zones on the foot.

Place the following points on the foot:

Pituitary gland

Lymphatics

Adrenal

7th Cervical

Large intestine

Thymus gland

Thyroid

Spine

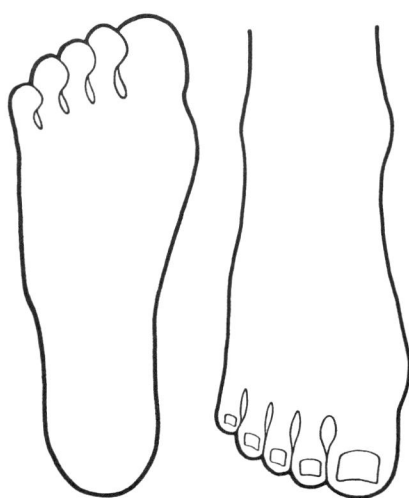

Name two functions of the pituitary gland.

_____

The four organs of elimination are:

_____

Name two functions of the thymus gland.

_____

_____

Where does digestion begin? _____

The lymph system consists of: _____

_____

What is the function of the parathyroid glands? _____

_____

What reflexes affect muscle tone and muscle strength? _____

_____

Assimilation is the job of the stomach. TRUE_____FALSE_____

The large intestine's job is to withdraw fluids and to return them to the system. TRUE_____FALSE_____

Name three reflexes to the knee. _____

Working the hand reflexes is as effective as working the foot reflexes.
TRUE_____FALSE_____

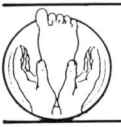

NOTE PAGE

Chapter 15
SYSTEMS OF THE BODY – RELATED REFLEXES

The following chapter will represent pictorially the systems of the body within the body and the foot.

Diagrams show the correlation between the locations of organs and glands in the body and on the foot. Below the diagrams are listed perhaps the most vital part of any Reflexology session – *OTHER AREAS INVOLVED.*

The body works as a *WHOLE.* No part stays dissassociated.

If you find a sensitive reflex, you may wish to check the associated areas since different organs work together to allow a functioning body.

Think of a car – a back wheel malalignment may cause the steering wheel to shimmy. A tiny misfire may cause the entire car to come to a halt.

The body is no different except that it is harder and more traumatic to get new spare parts when one of them malfunctions!

Therefore, become aware of nuances in the foot – notice relationships between organs, glands and structure.

There is a school of medicine that proposes that eye equilibrium is the most essential to the system's structure. In order to keep the eyes parallel to the ground, the entire structural anatomy may shift. Think how that affects the shoulders, spine, and therefore, certain nerves to certain organs.

Reread the functions of the organs to understand better how different parts work together – and try with your own creative intuition to understand why each area mentioned involves a relationship to the first one. This alone will make you an effective Reflexologist.

THE ENDOCRINE SYSTEM

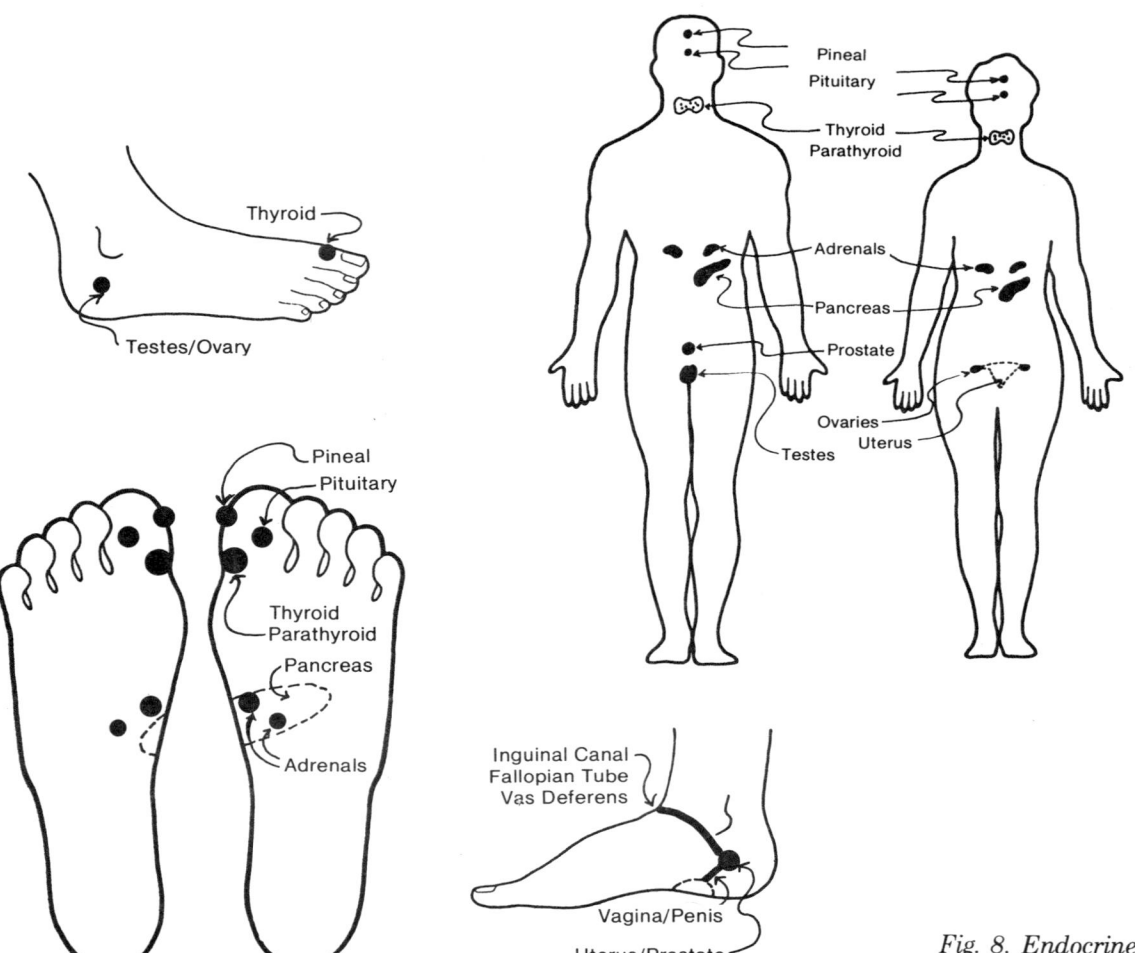

Fig. 8. Endocrine System

Other areas involved:

Pituitary	all endocrine glands, sex glands, entire nervous system, emotional balance, muscles, hypothalamus.
Pineal	muscular system, reproductive system, pain control, hypothalamus.
Thyroid	kidney, heart, all endocrine glands, hypothalamus, structural system, teeth.
Parathyroid	structural system, muscles, heart, teeth.
Adrenals	all endocrine glands, liver, heart, stomach, kidney, muscles, reproductive system, hypothalamus.
Sex organs **-testes/ovaries** **-prostate/uterus** **-vagina/penis**	all endocrine glands, particularly the pituitary gland, breast function, emotional balance, skin, nervous system; prostate/uterus relate to neck and cervical health; prostate relates to bladder; uterus depends on spine and large intestine health, neck and tonsils.
Pancreas	both endocrine and exocrine in function, related to all endocrine glands and to the entire digestive system, particularly adrenal gland, liver, stomach, common bile duct, duodenum.

THE LYMPHATIC AND CIRCULATORY SYSTEMS

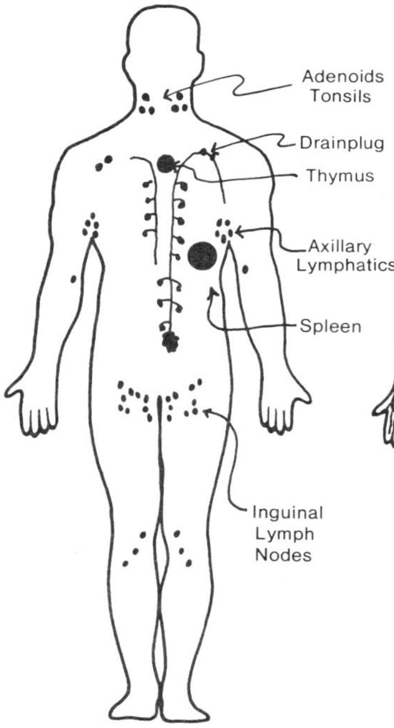

Lymphatic System

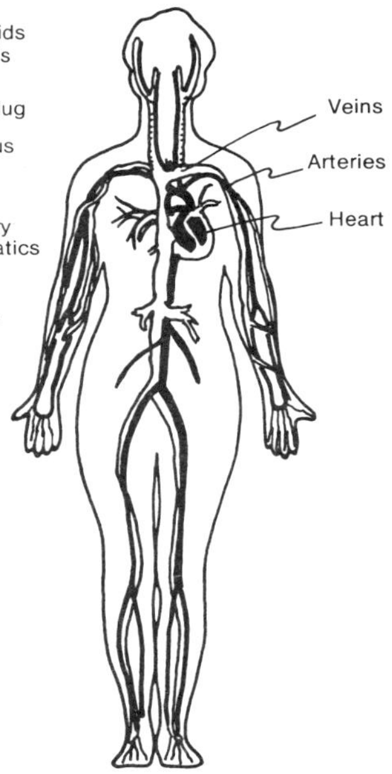

Circulatory System

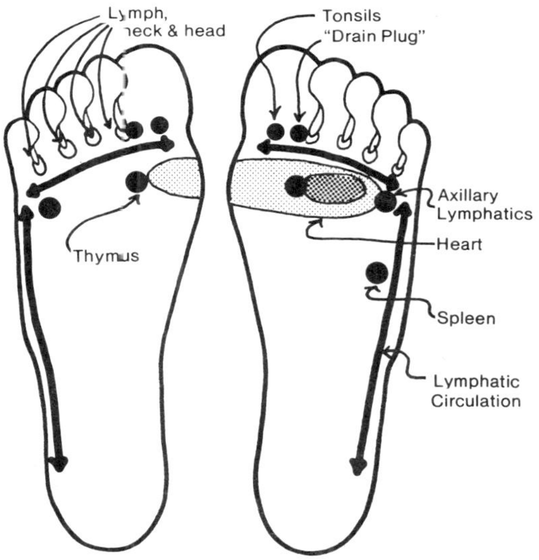

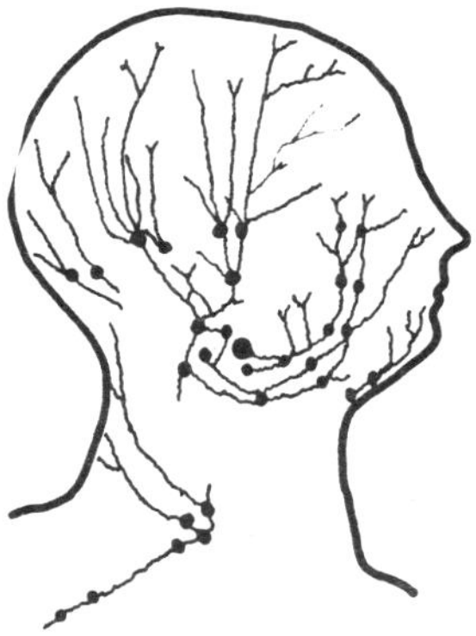

Major Lymph Nodes and Vessels in Head and Neck

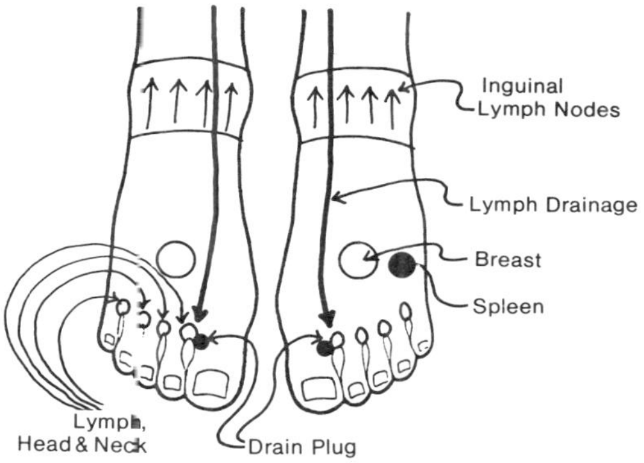

Fig. 9. Lymphatic and Circulatory Systems

Other areas involved:

Lymph nodes -head and neck -axillary, inguinal	blood vessels, cells, small intestine, kidney, circulatory system, drain plug, organs of elimination; lung kidney, skin, bowel.
Lymph/vessels	kidney, heart, adrenals, all areas affected by disease, small intestine, circulatory system, organs of elimination.
Thymus	defence of entire body, reacts to stress, therefore entire system and specifically adrenals, spleen, liver, lymph system.
Tonsils	neck, spine, bronchials, vagina, thymus, lymph nodes (all), drain plug.
Spleen	liver, heart, thymus, blood, lymph, large intestine.
Drain plug	lymph and blood circulation, kidney, heart, lymph nodes and vessels.
Heart	kidney, adrenals, blood circulation lungs, muscles, nerves, thyroid, pituitary, entire body.

THE RESPIRATORY SYSTEM

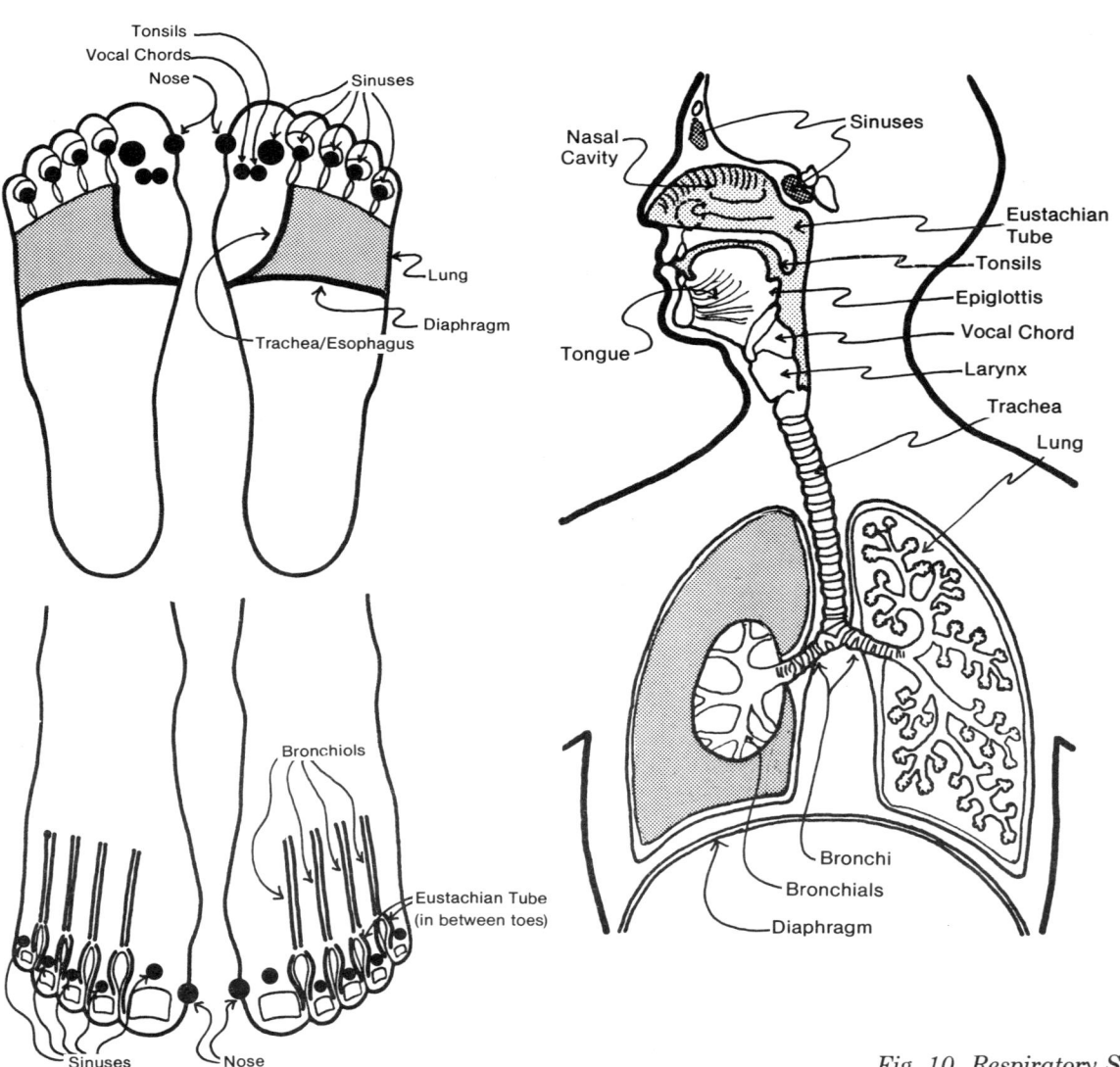

Fig. 10. Respiratory System

Other areas involved:

Nose	brain, stomach, lungs, sinuses, ileocecal valve, muscles.
Sinuses	mucous system, eyes, ears, head, eustachian tube, nose, intestines, stomach, ileocecal valve, gall bladder.
Trachea	sinuses, ileocecal, bronchials, vocal chords.
Bronchials	lungs, heart, adrenals, ileocecal valve, diaphragm, kidney, intestine.
Lungs	bronchials, heart, blood circulation, intestines, diaphragm, kidney, skin.
Diaphragm	lungs, heart, adrenals, pituitary, pineal, solar plexus, stomach.

THE DIGESTIVE SYSTEM

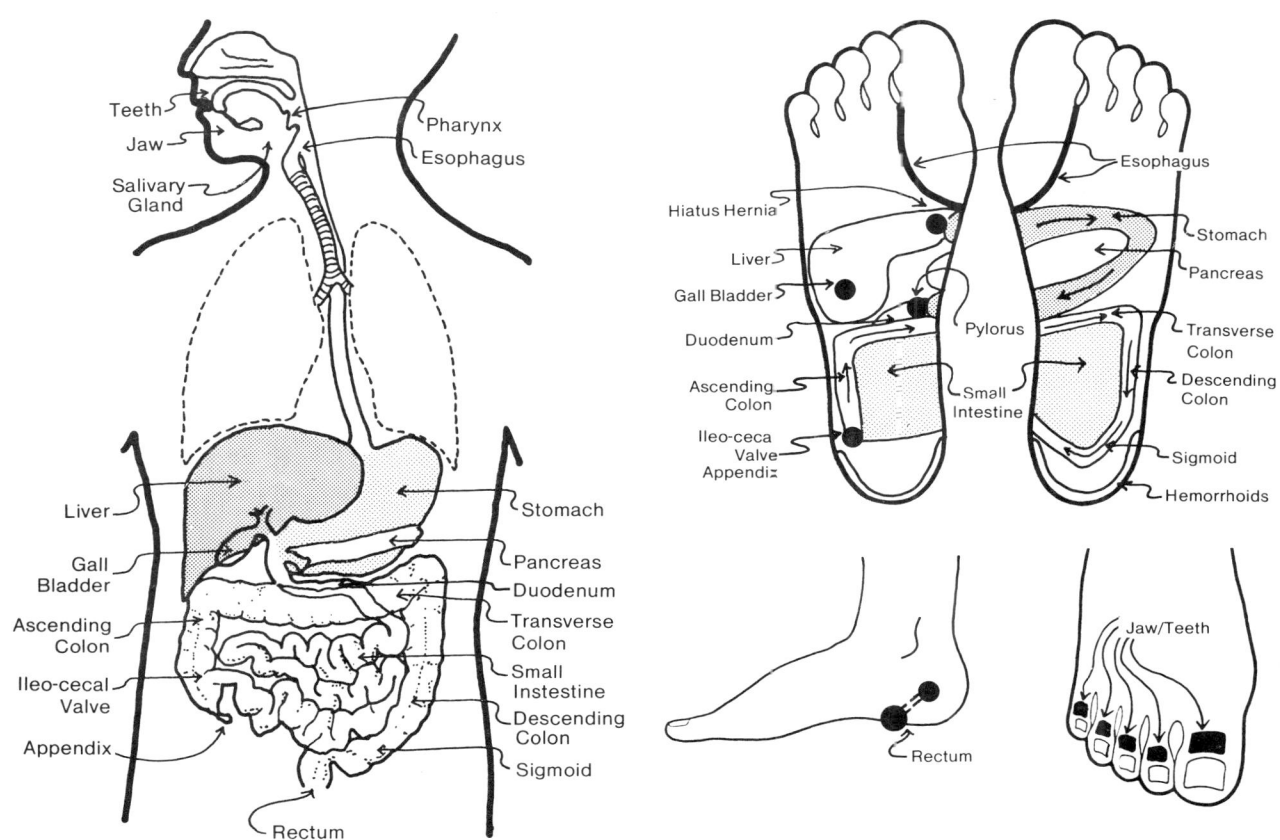

Fig. 11. Digestive System

Other areas involved:

Mouth	brain, teeth, stomach, salivary glands.
Teeth	neck, jaw, spine, sciatic, hip, shoulder.
Stomach	pituitary, thymus, adrenals, hypothalamus, diaphragm, small and large intestine, nervous system.
Pancreas	liver, gall bladder, small intestine, adrenals, stomach.
Liver	adrenals, pancreas, spleen, blood, veins, digestive system, sugar metabolism, filtering system, elimination, odour (skin).
Gall bladder	liver, spleen, small intestine, large intestine, pancreas, common bile duct.
Small intestine	assimilation of nutrients for cellular life, entire body.
Large intestine	organ of elimination, vitamin manufacturer, sinuses, ears, lungs, kidney, skin, health of body, involved in most disease.
Ileo-cecal valve	mucous system, sinuses, ears, nose, bronchials, large intestine.
Appendix	lymphatics, thymus, sinuses, large intestine, ileo-cecal valve.
Hemorrhoids	liver, prostate, large intestine, pancreas.
Hiatus hernia	stomach, diaphragm, solar plexus.
Rectum	prostate, large intestine, spine.

THE URINARY SYSTEM

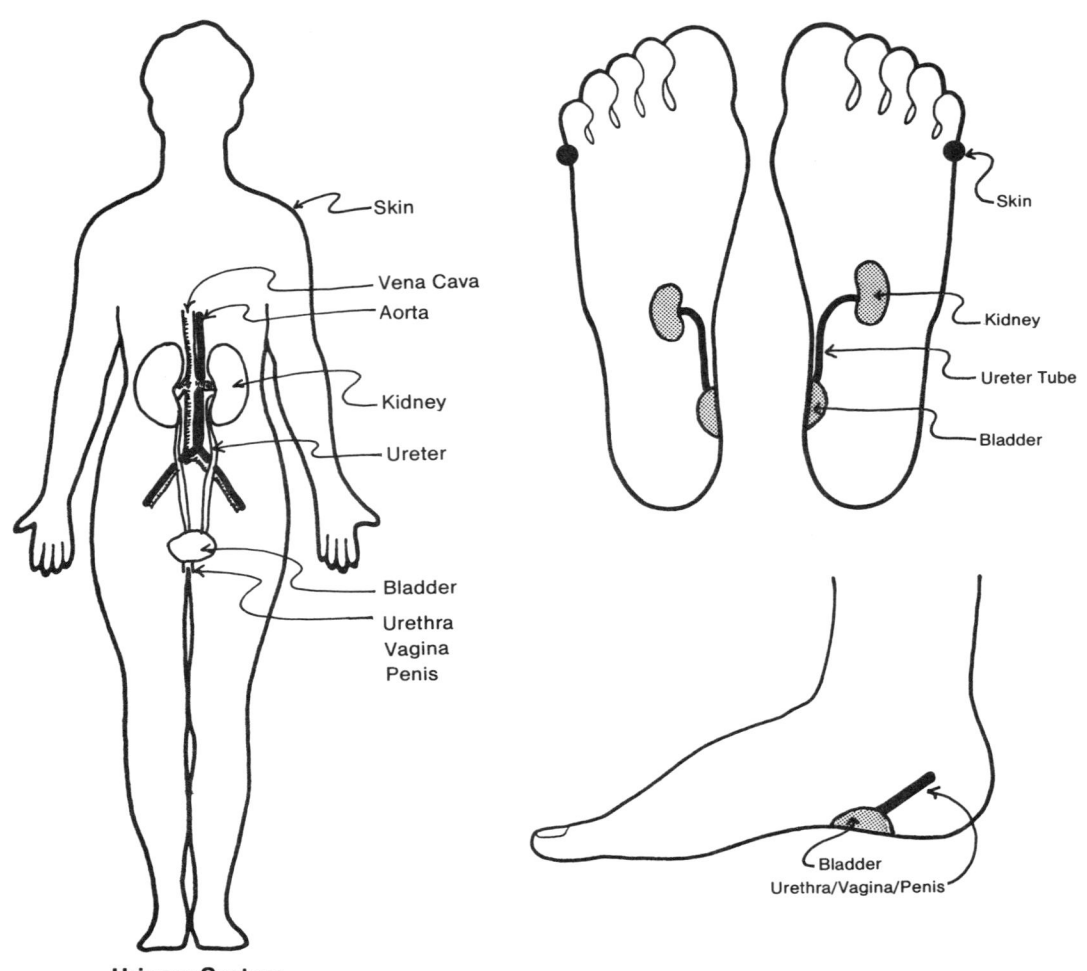

Urinary System

Fig. 12. Urinary System

Skin
Vena Cava
Aorta
Kidney
Ureter
Bladder
Urethra
Vagina
Penis

Skin
Kidney
Ureter Tube
Bladder

Bladder
Urethra/Vagina/Penis

Other areas involved:

Kidney	organ of elimination; adrenal, heart, blood pressure, pituitary, thyroid, lymph, parathyroid, skin, large intestine, lungs.
Ureter tube	kidney, bladder, parathyroid, urethra, prostate.
Bladder	pineal, kidney, thymus, adrenals, parathyroid, urethra, prostate.
Urethra	penis, vagina, kidney, bladder, prostate, ureter tube.
Skin	organ of elimination; affects and is affected by organs below any given area and by organs of elimination. Lung, kidney, large intestine.

THE STRUCTURAL SYSTEM, THE NERVOUS SYSTEM AND SENSORY ORGANS

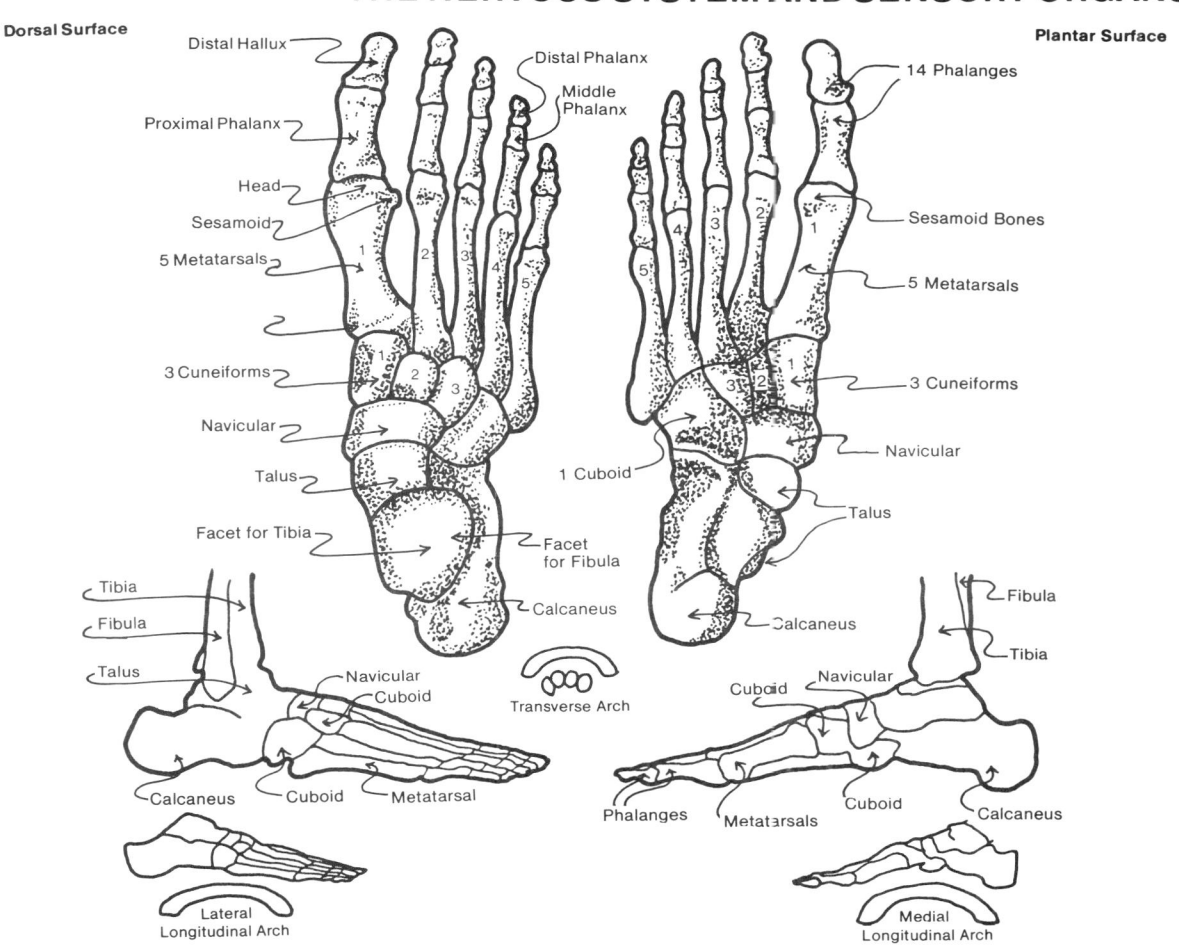

Fig. 13. Skeletal Structure of Foot

Other areas involved:

Spine	entire body – all organs, all muscles, nerves, brain.
7th cervical, neck	body tension, gall bladder, prostate, uterus, arm function (tingling or numb), eyes, ears, relaxation point, for points above waist.
Coccyx	body tension, eyes, relaxation point. for points below waist.
Shoulder	gall bladder, pancreas, 7th cervical, sciatic, teeth, hip, sacrum.
Hip	shoulder, spine, sciatic nerve, foot.
Knee	elbow, hip, spine, foot.
Solar plexus	key relaxation point, entire body – all functions.
Back muscles	hold up spine on either side and affect and are affected by abdominal muscles.
Buttocks	legs, hip, sacrum, low back.
Eyes	kidney, 7th cervical, coccyx, shoulder lymphatics.
Ears	large intestine, ileo-cecal valve, cervicals, 7th cervical, coccyx, shoulder lymphatics.

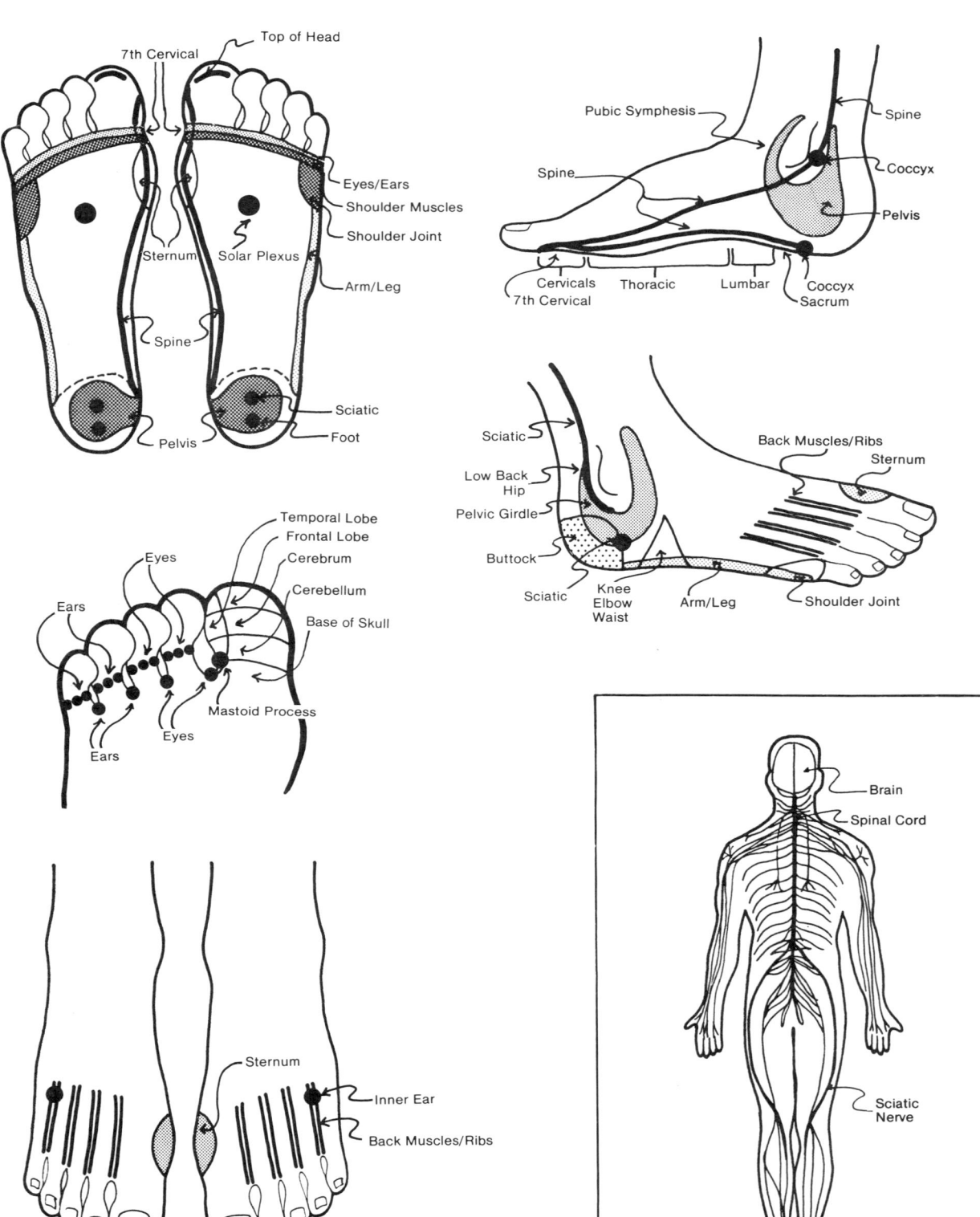

Fig. 14. Foot Reflexes for Structural, Nervous and Sensory Systems

Fig. 15. Peripheral Nervous System

Musculature - Frontal

Musculature – Back

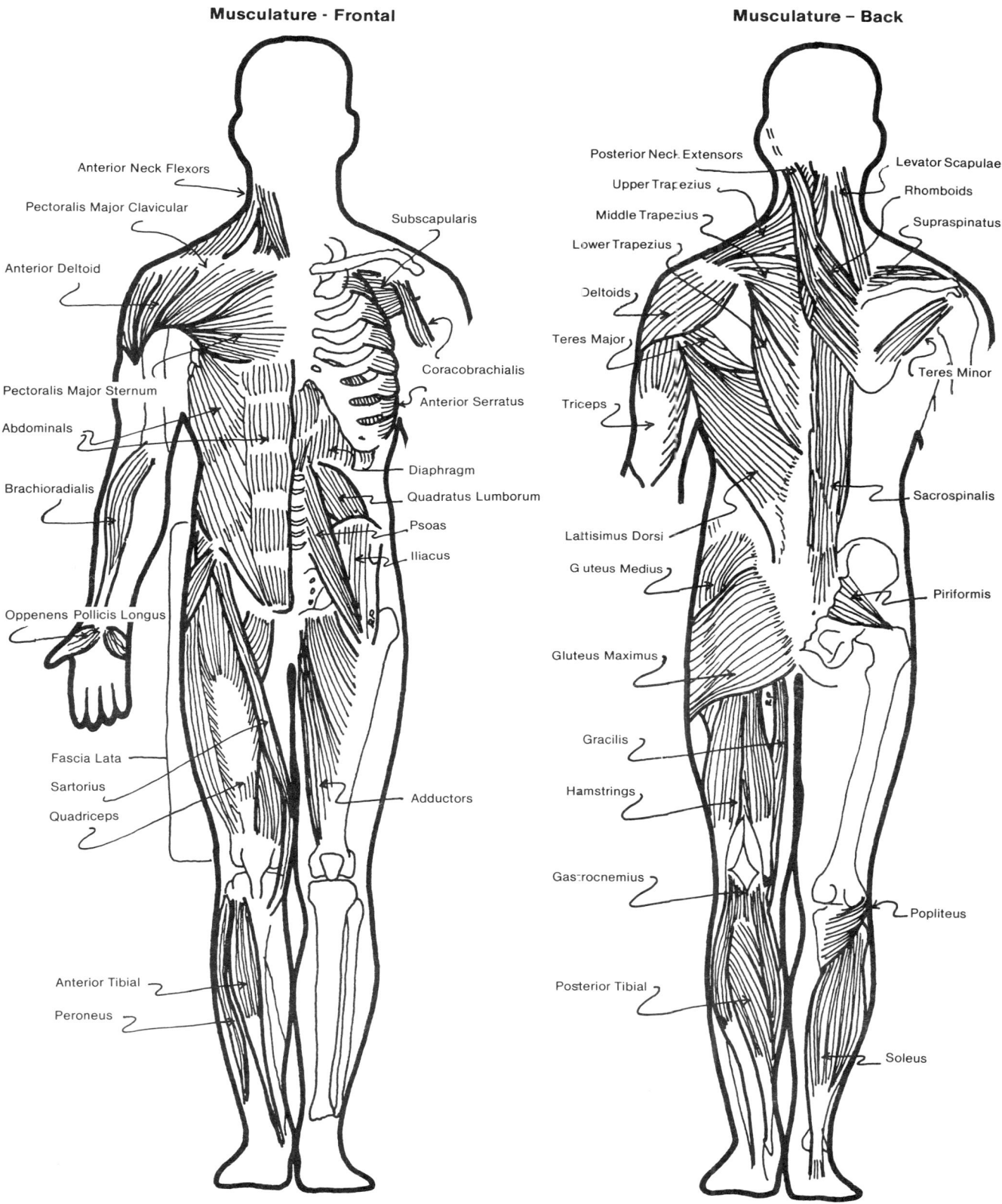

Anterior Neck Flexors

Pectoralis Major Clavicular

Anterior Deltoid

Pectoralis Major Sternum

Abdominals

Brachioradialis

Oppenens Pollicis Longus

Fascia Lata

Sartorius

Quadriceps

Anterior Tibial

Peroneus

Subscapularis

Coracobrachialis

Anterior Serratus

Diaphragm

Quadratus Lumborum

Psoas

Iliacus

Adductors

Posterior Neck Extensors

Upper Trapezius

Middle Trapezius

Lower Trapezius

Deltoids

Teres Major

Triceps

Lattisimus Dorsi

Gluteus Medius

Gluteus Maximus

Gracilis

Hamstrings

Gastrocnemius

Posterior Tibial

Levator Scapulae

Rhomboids

Supraspinatus

Teres Minor

Sacrospinalis

Piriformis

Popliteus

Soleus

Fig. 16. Musculature of the Body

93

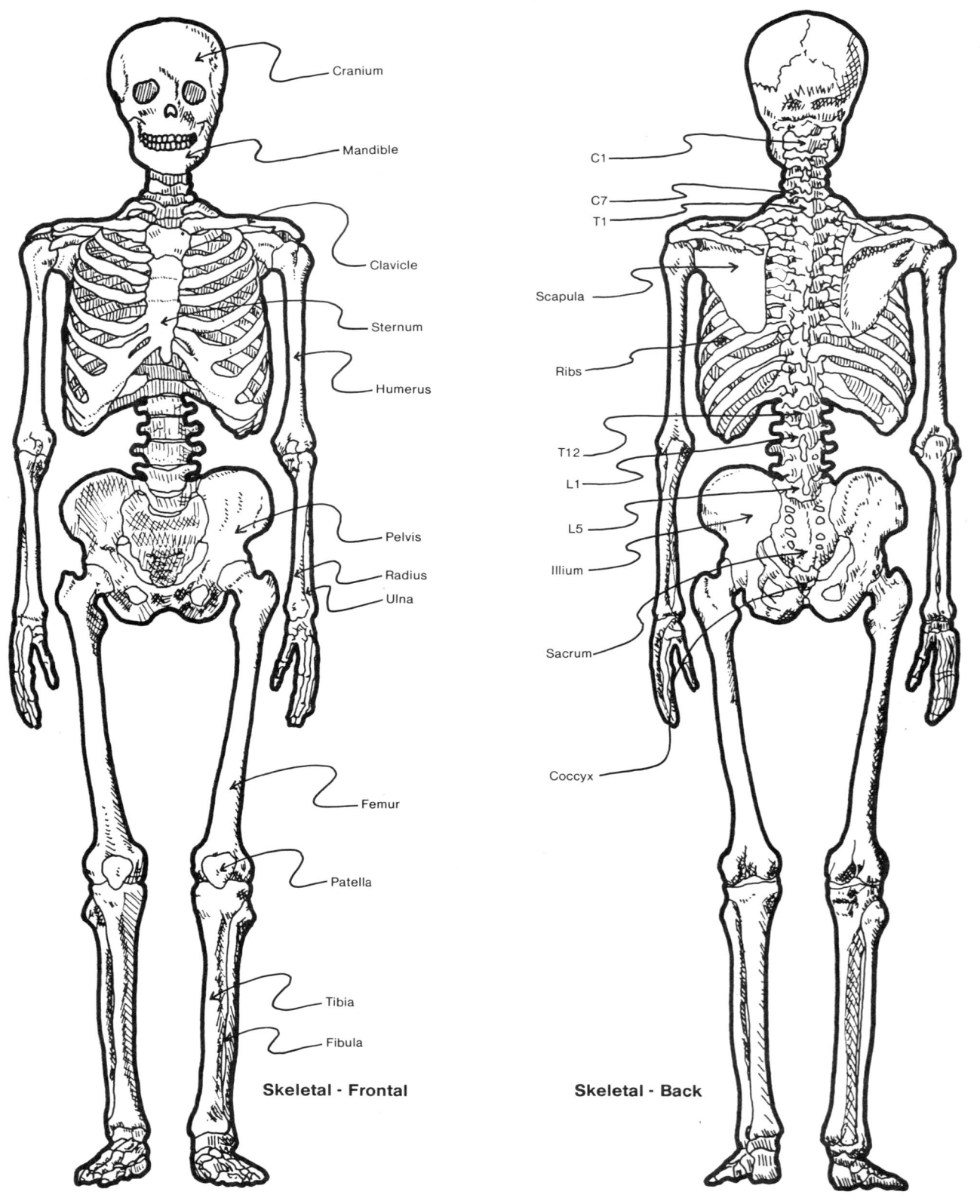

Cranium

Mandible

Clavicle

Sternum

Humerus

Pelvis

Radius

Ulna

Femur

Patella

Tibia

Fibula

Skeletal - Frontal

C1

C7

T1

Scapula

Ribs

T12

L1

L5

Illium

Sacrum

Coccyx

Skeletal - Back

Fig. 17. Skeletal Structure of the Body

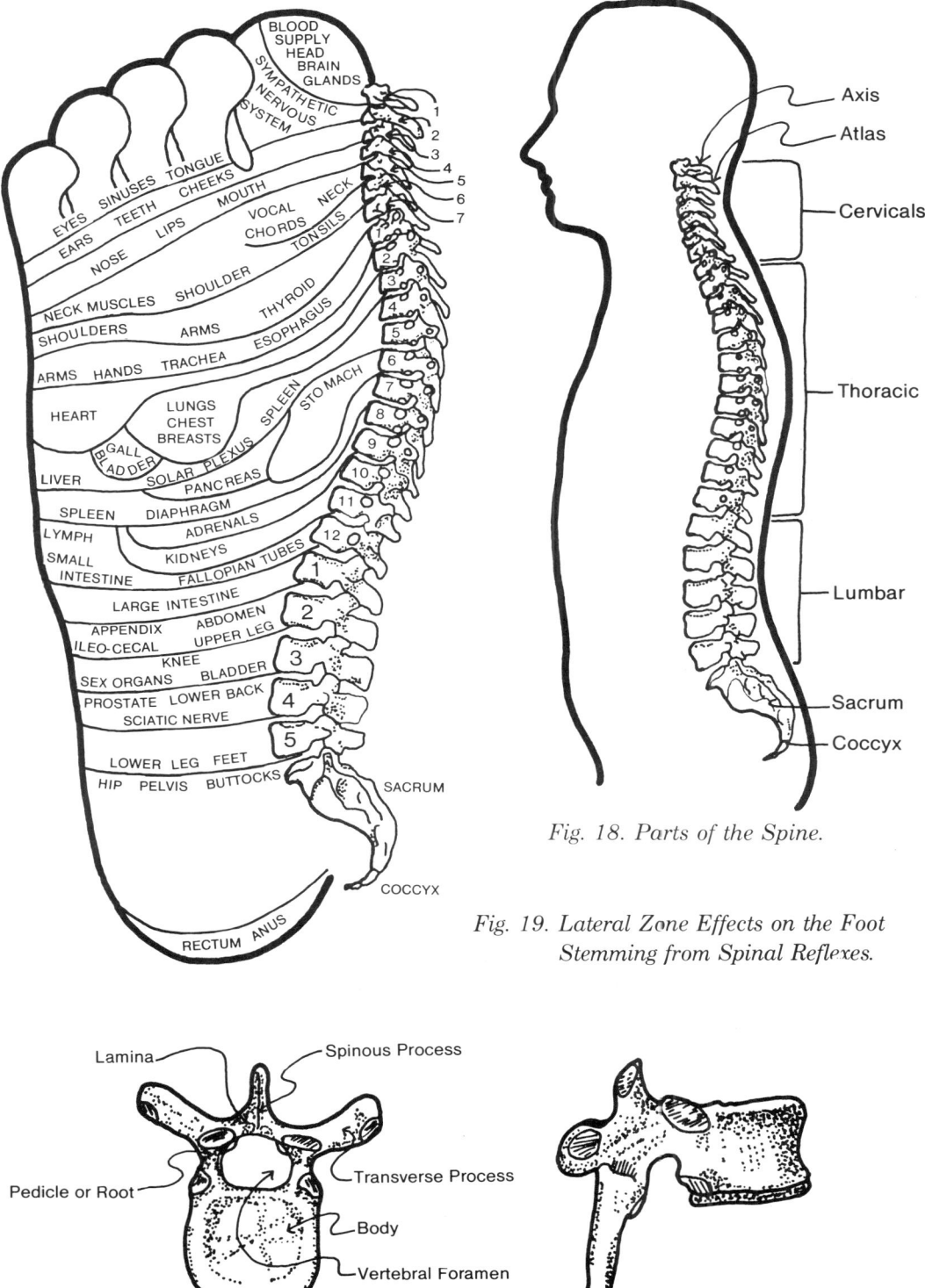

Fig. 18. Parts of the Spine.

Fig. 19. Lateral Zone Effects on the Foot Stemming from Spinal Reflexes.

Fig. 20. A Thoracic Vertebrae, Superior and Lateral View.

FOOT CHART

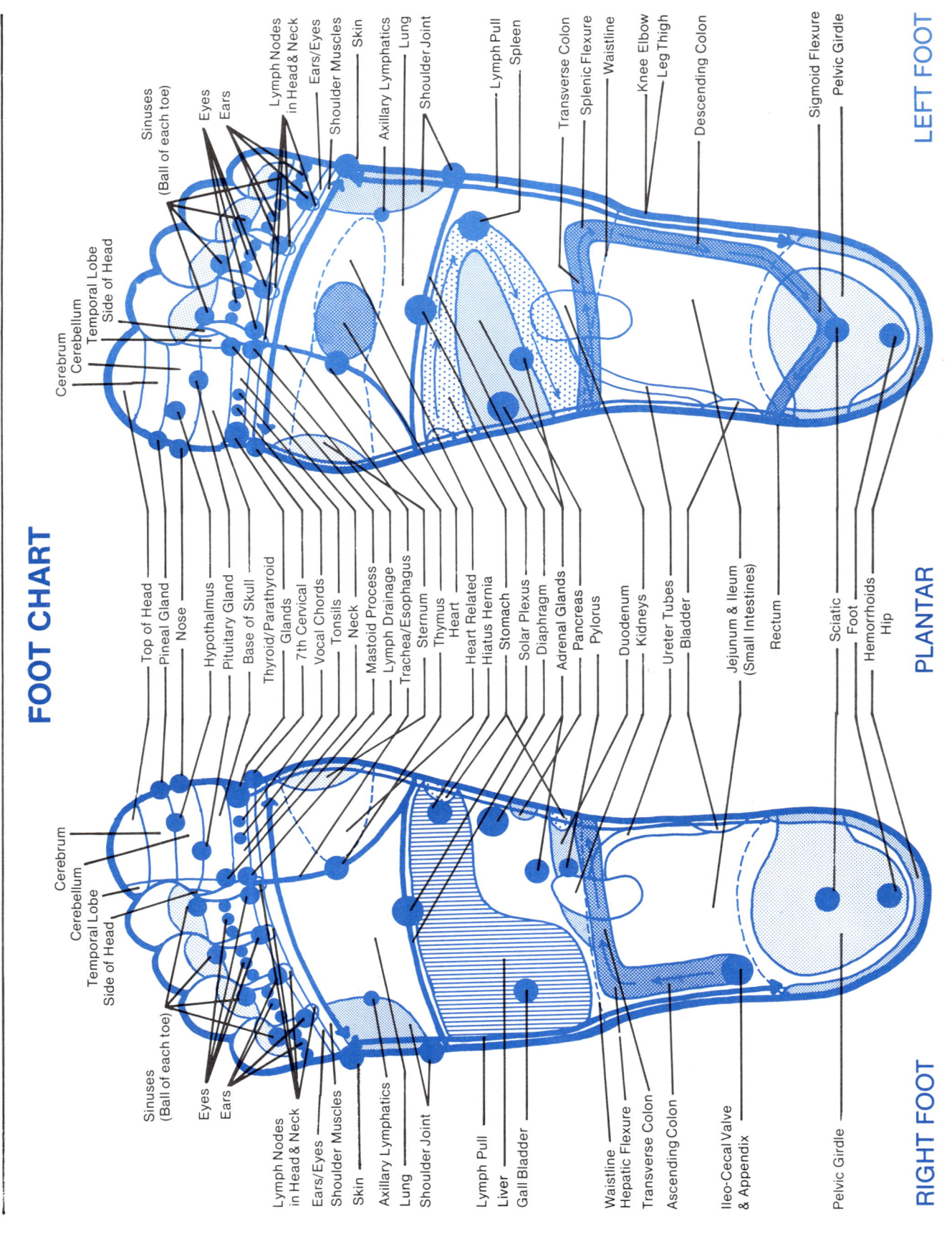

LEFT FOOT

PLANTAR

RIGHT FOOT

Left foot labels:
Sinuses (Ball of each toe)
Eyes
Ears
Lymph Nodes in Head & Neck
Ears/Eyes
Shoulder Muscles
Skin
Axillary Lymphatics
Lung
Shoulder Joint
Lymph Pull
Spleen
Transverse Colon
Splenic Flexure
Waistline
Knee Elbow
Leg Thigh
Descending Colon
Sigmoid Flexure
Pelvic Girdle

Cerebrum
Cerebellum
Temporal Lobe
Side of Head

Top of Head
Pineal Gland
Nose
Hypothalmus
Pituitary Gland
Base of Skull
Thyroid/Parathyroid Glands
7th Cervical
Vocal Chords
Tonsils
Neck
Mastoid Process
Lymph Drainage
Trachea/Esophagus
Sternum
Thymus
Heart
Heart Related
Hiatus Hernia
Stomach
Solar Plexus
Diaphragm
Adrenal Glands
Pancreas
Pylorus
Duodenum
Kidneys
Ureter Tubes
Bladder
Jejunum & Ileum (Small Intestines)
Rectum
Sciatic
Foot
Hemorrhoids
Hip

Right foot labels:
Cerebrum
Cerebellum
Temporal Lobe
Side of Head

Sinuses (Ball of each toe)
Eyes
Ears
Lymph Nodes in Head & Neck
Ears/Eyes
Shoulder Muscles
Skin
Axillary Lymphatics
Lung
Shoulder Joint
Lymph Pull
Liver
Gall Bladder
Waistline
Hepatic Flexure
Transverse Colon
Ascending Colon
Ileo-Cecal Valve & Appendix
Pelvic Girdle

96

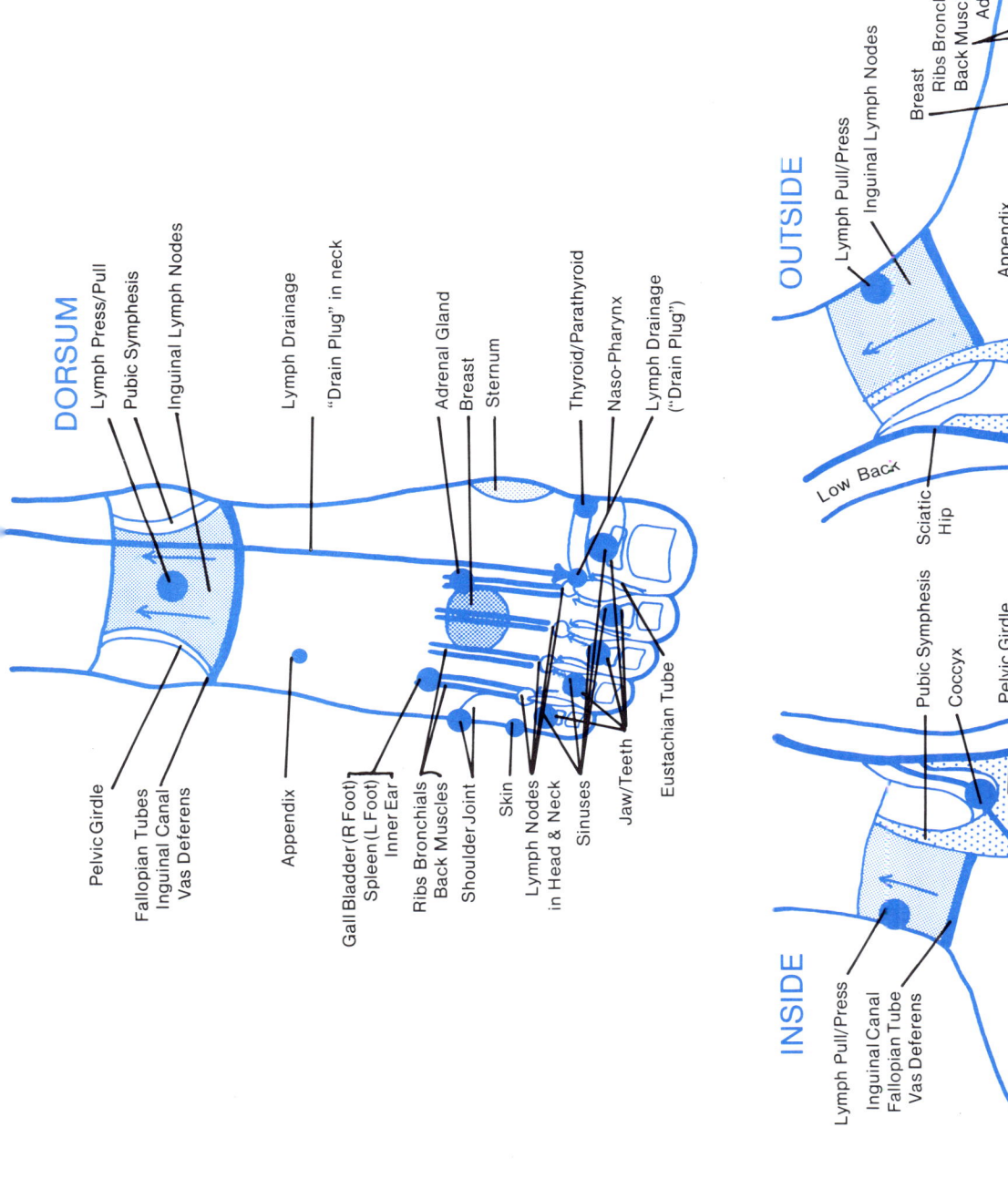

DORSUM

Lymph Press/Pull
Pubic Symphesis
Inguinal Lymph Nodes

Lymph Drainage
"Drain Plug" in neck

Adrenal Gland
Breast
Sternum

Thyroid/Parathyroid
Naso-Pharynx
Lymph Drainage
("Drain Plug")

Pelvic Girdle

Fallopian Tubes
Inguinal Canal
Vas Deferens

Appendix

Gall Bladder (R Foot)
Spleen (L Foot)
Inner Ear

Ribs Bronchials
Back Muscles
Shoulder Joint
Skin
Lymph Nodes
in Head & Neck
Sinuses
Jaw/Teeth
Eustachian Tube

OUTSIDE

Lymph Pull/Press
Inguinal Lymph Nodes

Breast
Ribs Bronchials
Back Muscles
Adrenal Gland

Sedation Point

Inner Ear

Shoulder Joint

Appendix

Arm
Leg

Waist Elbow Knee
Low Back

Low Back

Sciatic
Hip

Pelvic Girdle
Ovary Testes

Buttock

INSIDE

Lymph Pull/Press
Inguinal Canal
Fallopian Tube
Vas Deferens

Pubic Symphesis
Coccyx

Pelvic Girdle

Prostate
uterus
Rectum

Vagina Urethra
Penis

Bladder

Sacrum
Coccyx

Lumbar

Thoracic

S P I N E

S P I N E

Sternum

Neck

Pineal Gland
Nose
Top of Head
7th Cervical

Fig. 21. Foot Reflexology Chart

97

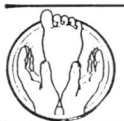

Chapter 16
THE COLOURING BOOK – THE BODY AND THE FOOT

Visualize Your Organs

On the outline of the body, place all the organs mentioned in the last few pages. Colour them in by systems:

RESPIRATORY - Orange; ENDOCRINE - Yellow; CIRCULATORY - Red; DIGESTIVE - Purple; LYMPHATIC - Blue; NERVOUS - Pink; SKELE-TAL STRUCTURAL - Brown; URINARY - Green; SENSORY - White.

MAKE NOTE OF THE FOUR ORGANS OF ELIMINATION:

_____, _____
_____, _____

Draw black or blue lines through those organs.

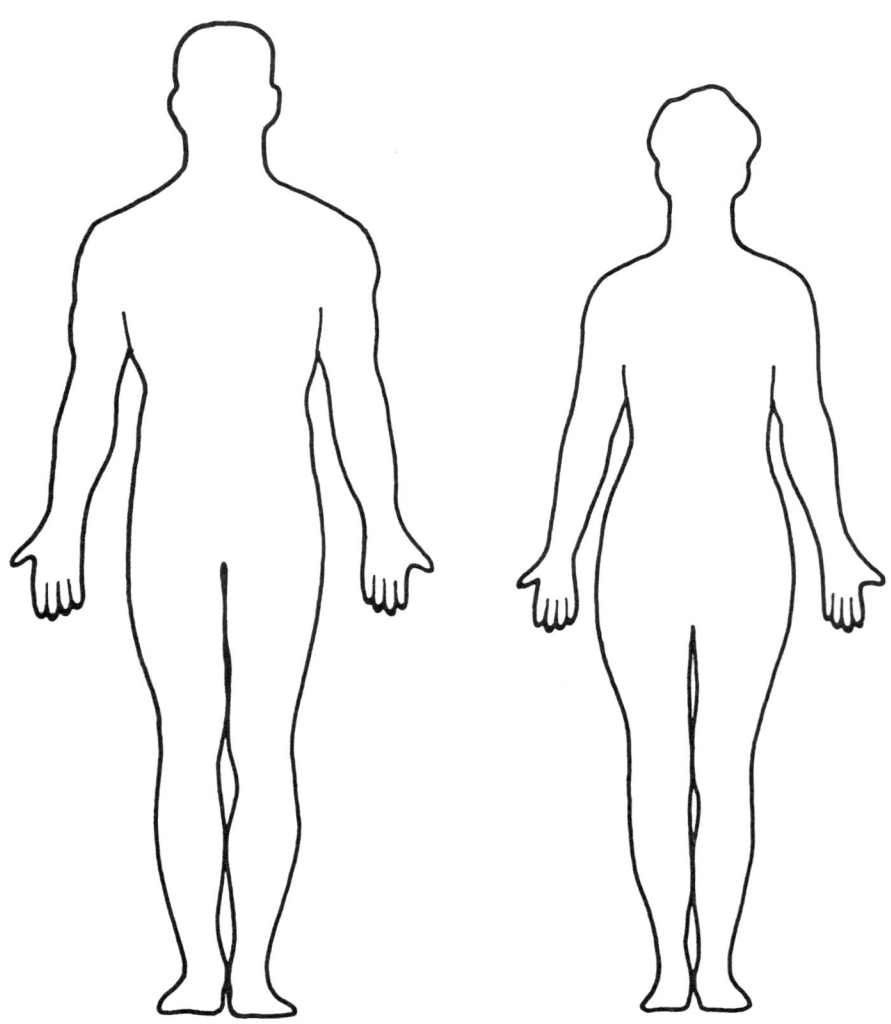

Understand the Foot

Place reflexes to various organs on the feet. Colour them in by system according to the colour code on the body.

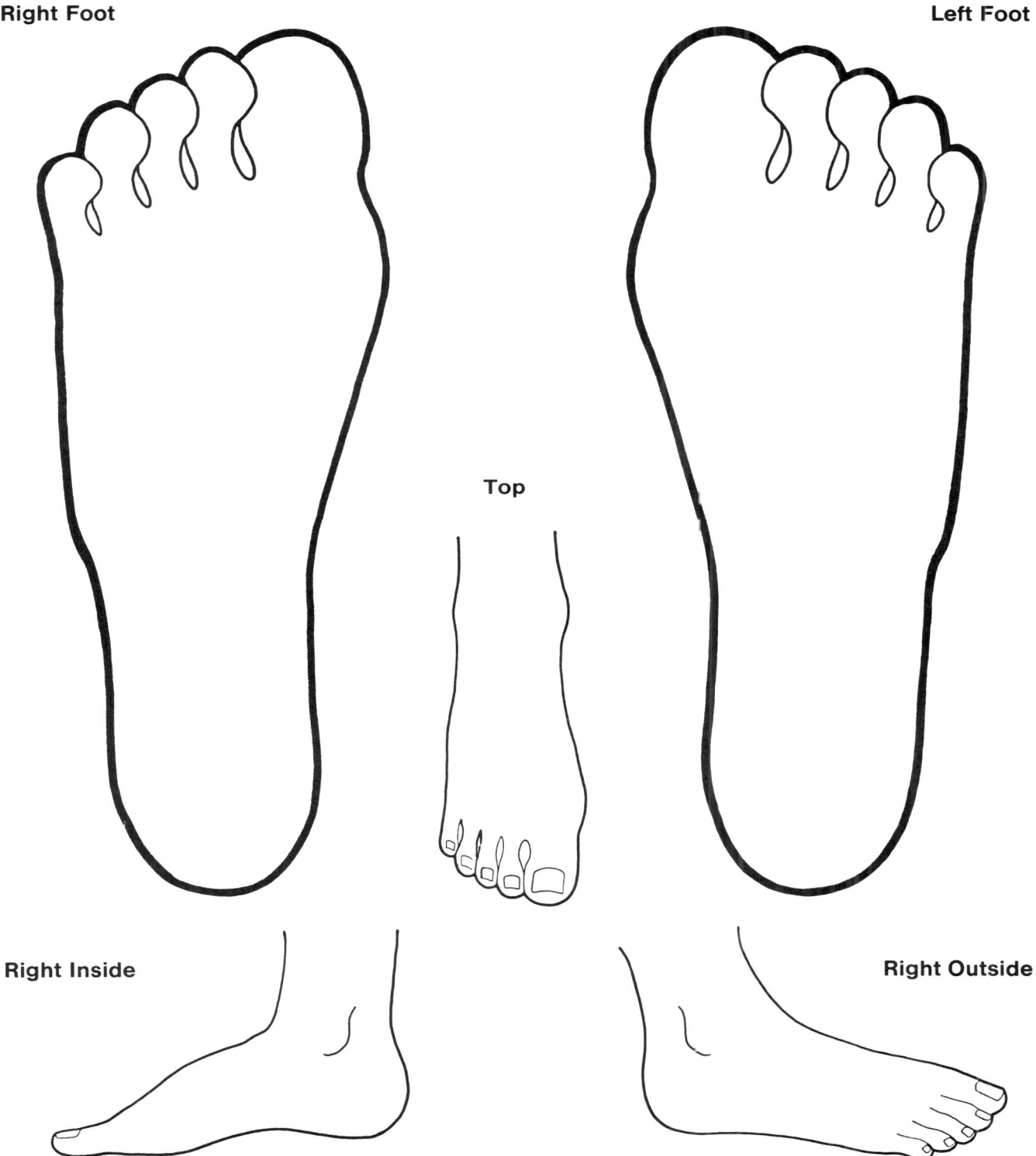

Right Foot

Left Foot

Top

Right Inside

Right Outside

Foot Chart
Name the reflexes.

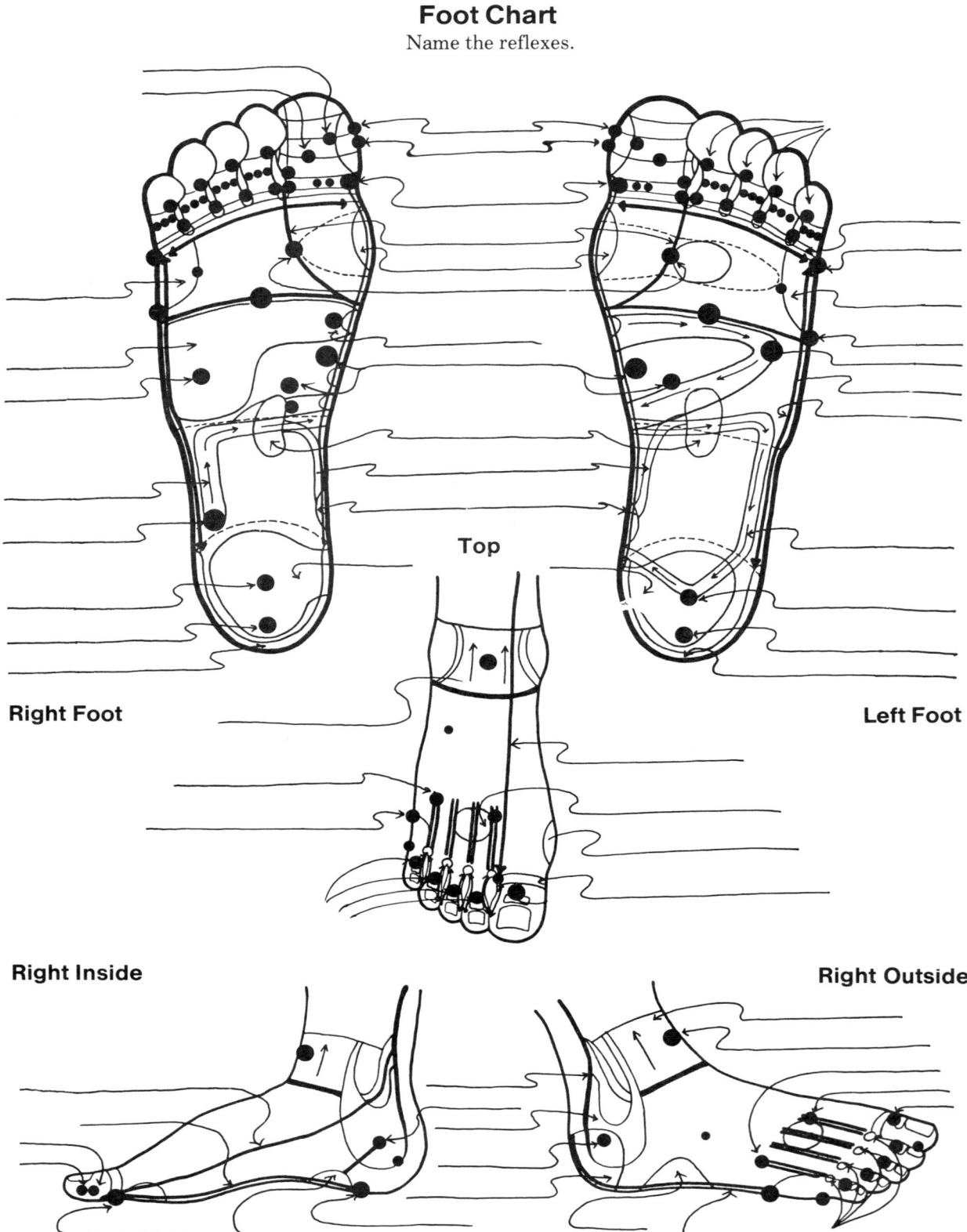

Top

Right Foot

Left Foot

Right Inside

Right Outside

Foot Chart
Draw in the reflexes.

Right Foot

Left Foot

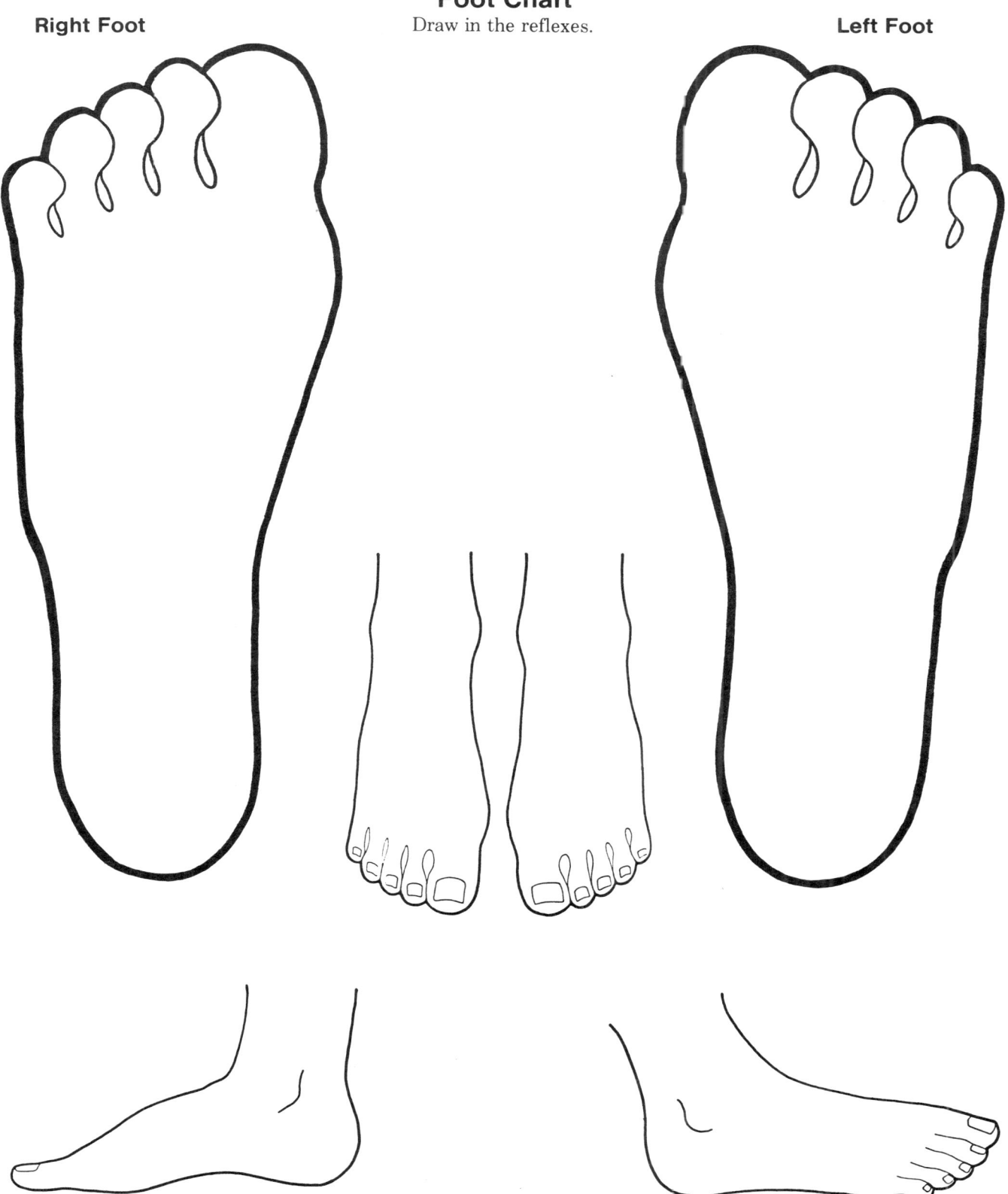

Understand the Foot

Draw in and colour the reflexes on the foot. Yes, the drawing is upside down.

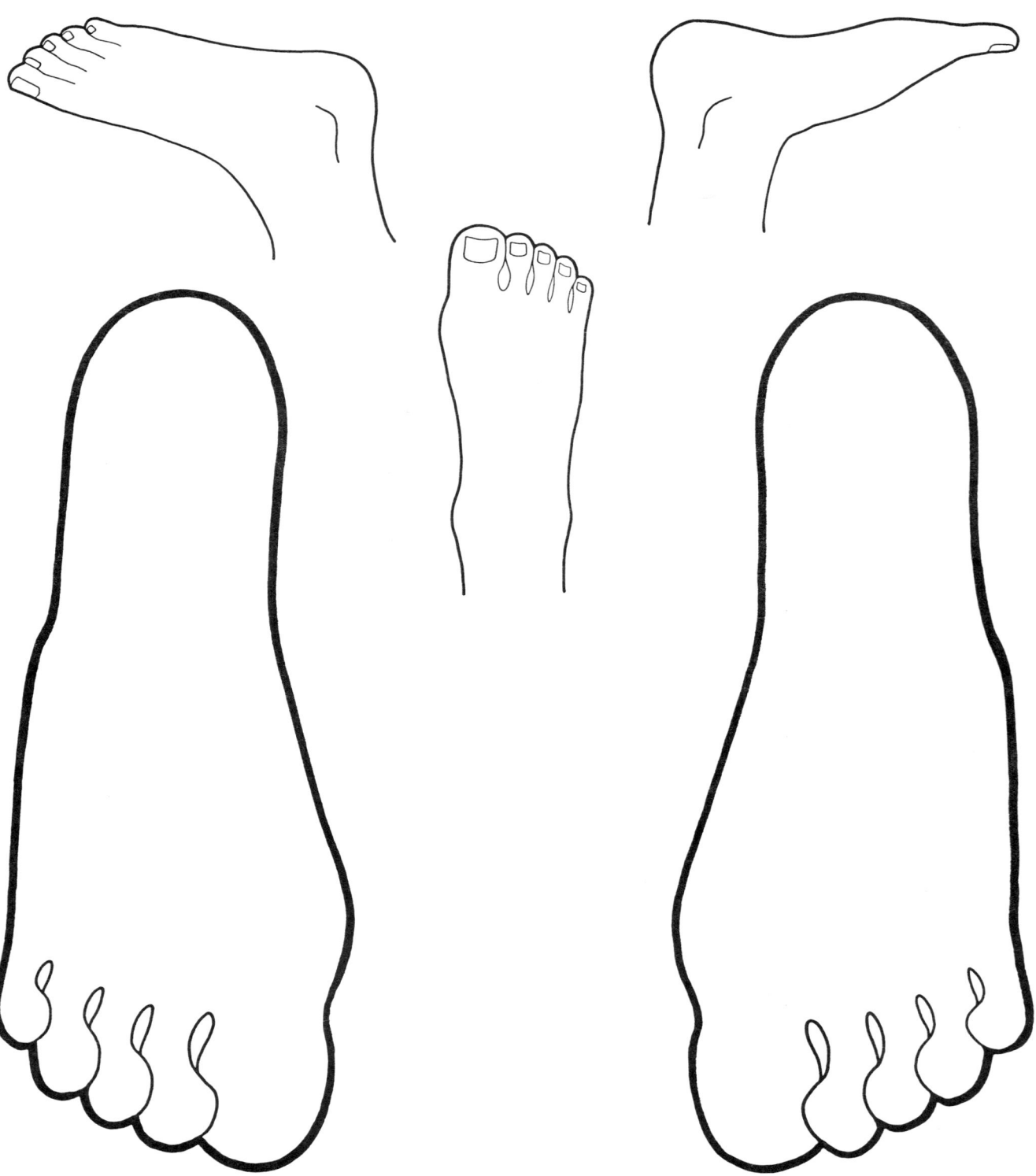

Knowing the Foot

Compare right and left foot.

What reflexes are in the right foot only?_____

_____

What reflexes are in the left foot only? _____

_____

What reflexes in what foot do not touch the ground when you walk? _____

_____

What reflexes are on the side of the foot, big toe side? _____

_____

What reflexes are on the pinky toe side? _____

_____

Which organs or parts of the body have more than one reflex on the foot? _____

Draw the answers in:

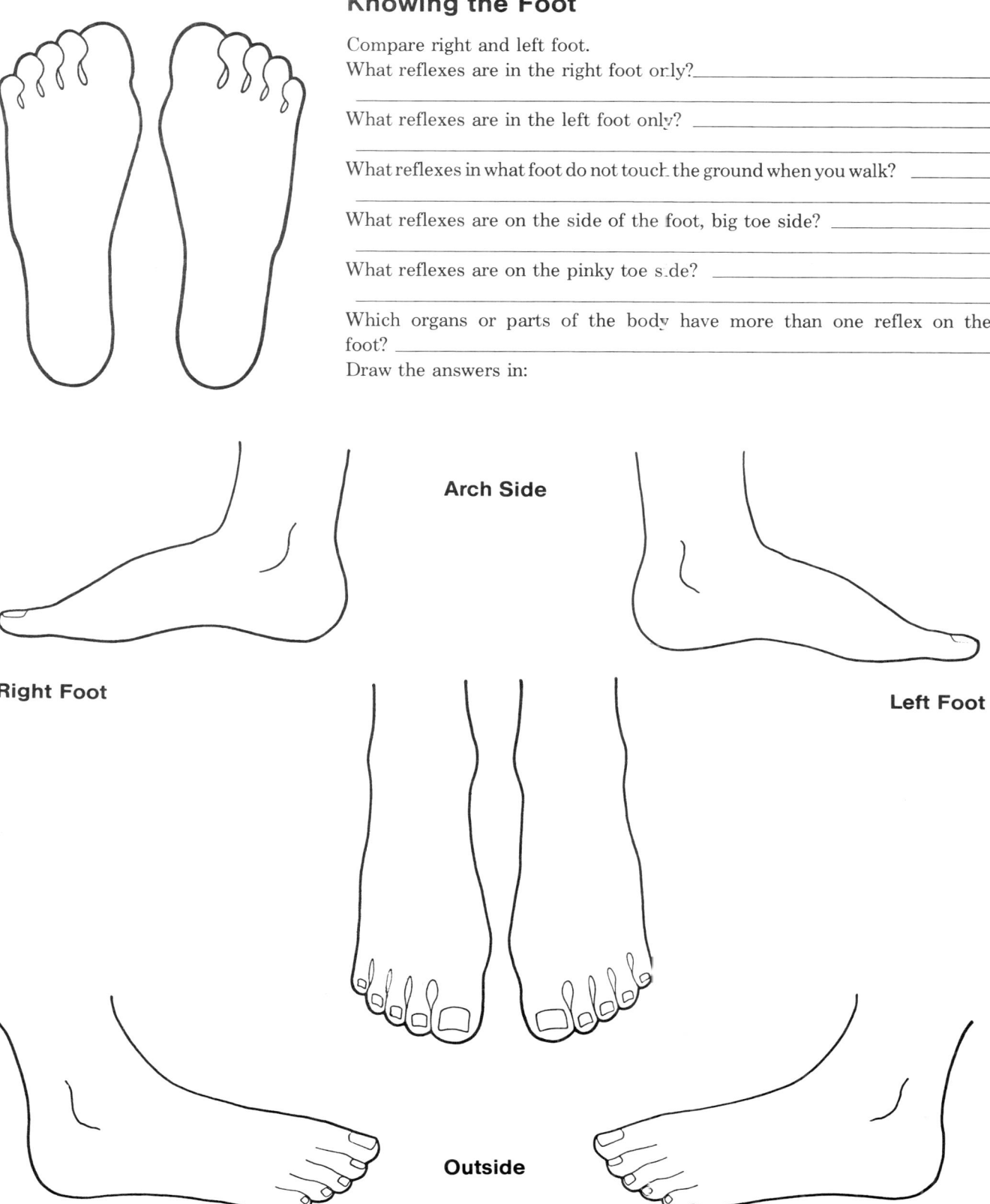

Arch Side

Right Foot

Left Foot

Outside

103

The Hand Reflexology Chart

For reflexes not indicated, survey the foot chart, note the similarities and differences and apply your knowledge to determine the location of the foot reflex in the hand.

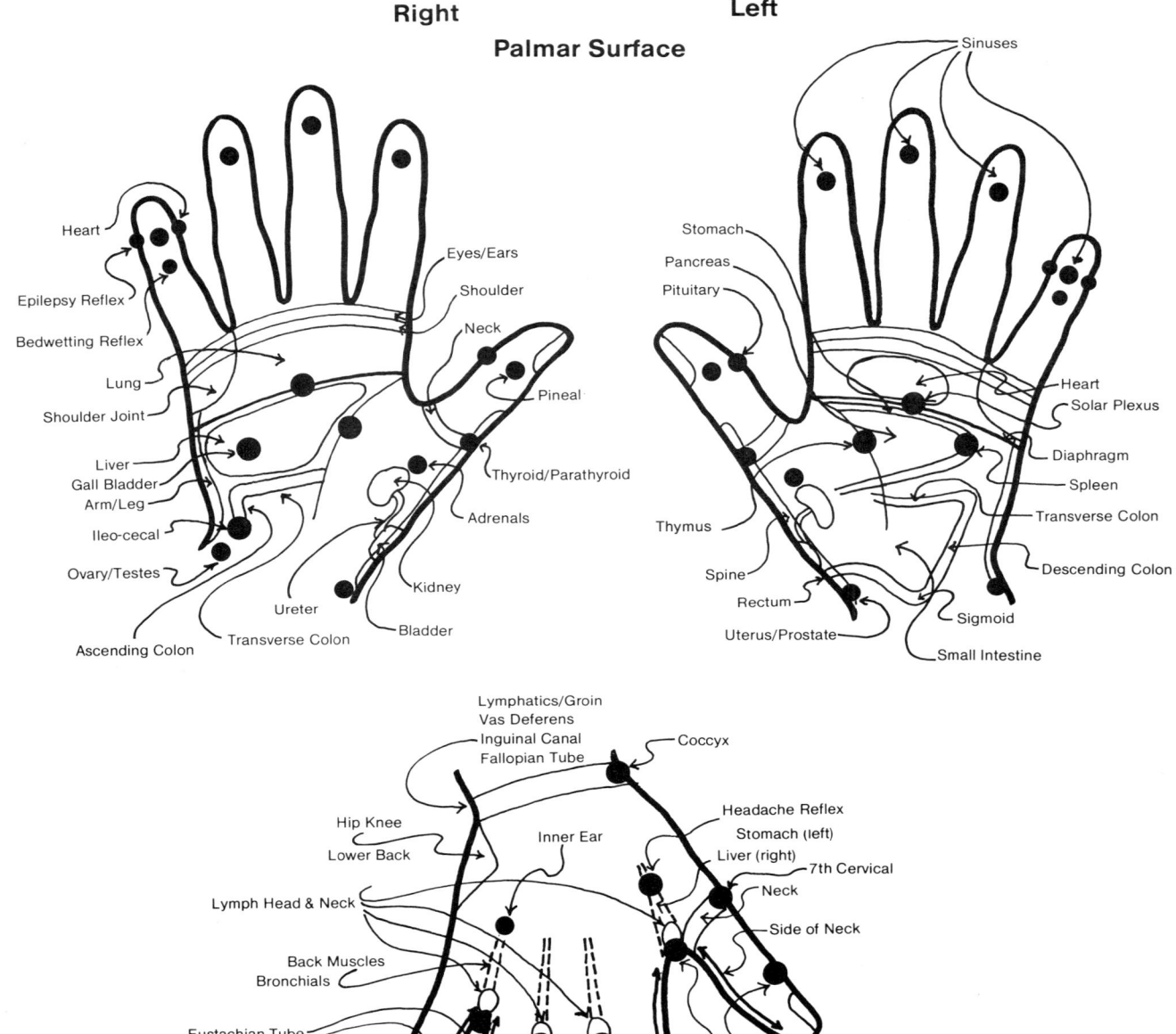

Right

Palmar Surface

Heart

Epilepsy Reflex

Bedwetting Reflex

Lung

Shoulder Joint

Liver

Gall Bladder

Arm/Leg

Ileo-cecal

Ovary/Testes

Ascending Colon

Transverse Colon

Eyes/Ears

Shoulder

Neck

Pineal

Thyroid/Parathyroid

Adrenals

Kidney

Ureter

Bladder

Left

Sinuses

Stomach

Pancreas

Pituitary

Thymus

Spine

Rectum

Uterus/Prostate

Heart

Solar Plexus

Diaphragm

Spleen

Transverse Colon

Descending Colon

Sigmoid

Small Intestine

Lymphatics/Groin
Vas Deferens
Inguinal Canal
Fallopian Tube

Coccyx

Hip Knee

Lower Back

Inner Ear

Headache Reflex

Stomach (left)

Liver (right)

7th Cervical

Neck

Side of Neck

Lymph Head & Neck

Back Muscles

Bronchials

Eustachian Tube

Jaw/Teeth

Eyes/Ears

Teeth

Dorsal Surface

Fig. 22. Hand Reflexology Chart

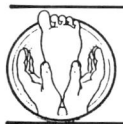

NOTE PAGE

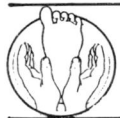

Chapter 17
SOME DISCOMFORTS AND THEIR MAJOR REFLEXES

Always work the entire foot. Sometimes it is necessary to pay particular attention to specific reflexes to get to the major causes of dis-ease. This chapter deals with those specific reflexes that you might address yourself to.

CONDITION	MAJOR REFLEXES TO BE WORKED
Alcoholism	Pituitary, adrenals, pancreas, pineal, liver.
Allergies	Adrenals, stomach, large intestine, liver, thymus.
Anemia	Spleen, liver.
Arthritis	Parathyroids, adrenals, stomach, small and large intestine, pituitary, kidneys, thyroid.
Back pain	Spine, hip, pelvis (work in same rhythm as breathing).
Burping	Sigmoid flexure, stomach, esophagus, diaphragm.
Bursitis	Kidneys, shoulder joint, adrenals, parathyroids, thymus.
Car sickness	Sinuses, 4th toe, 4th finger, 7th cervical, base of 4th finger and toe, webbing between thumb and first finger, stroke the back of the nails up the back of the hand.
Cataracts	Eyes, kidneys, colon, coccyx, 7th cervical, shoulders.
Cold feet	Pancreas, whole foot for circulation.
Colds	Top of toes and fingers, lung, bronchials, kidneys, ileo-cecal valve.
Colitis	Small and large intestine, solar plexus.
Constipation	Solar plexus, sigmoid flexure, ileo-cecal valve, liver, gall bladder, adrenals, coccyx, prostate, uterus, spine, large intestine, spleen.
Convulsions	Big and little toe pads, top of the head, heart, spleen, lymph, liver, intestines, spine, coccyx, sex glands.
Crohns disease	Same as colitis.
Depression	Head, kidneys, adrenals, neck, solar plexus, pylorus, ileo-cecal valve.
Diabetes	Pancreas, liver adrenals, stomach, thyroid, pituitary.
Diarrhea	Small and large intestine, ileo-cecal valve, stomach, gall bladder, liver, spleen.
Dizziness	Inner ear, neck, liver, balance point (between 5th and 4th toes in between the tendons).
Dry skin	Adrenals, kidneys, skin, thyroid, liver, dry-brush massage.
Ear problems	Ear, inner ear, tonsils, eustachian tube, lymphatics, neck, ileo-cecal valve, large intestine, 4th and 5th fingers and toes, on and between.
Eczema	Kidneys, skin, solar plexus, adrenals, thymus, 7th cervical-coccyx.
Edema	Lymph system, adrenals, heart, kidneys, drain plug.
Emphysema	Lungs, bronchials, sinus, adrenals, ileo-cecal valve, solar plexus, kidneys.
Epilepsy	Kidneys, 7th cervical, colon, liver, spine, head, pituitary.
Extreme sensitivity	Solar plexus.

Extreme sensitivity to the solar plexus may indicate heart condition.

Fainting	Pituitary.
Fatigue	Pituitary, liver, adrenals, tap the thymus on the sternum below clavicle.
Female disorders	Ovaries, uterus, pituitary, adrenals, thyroid, pineal.
Fluid retention	Lymphatic system, *drain plug*, see *Edema*.
Foot odour	Kidneys, liver, adrenals, skin.
Gall bladder	
Gall stones	Gall bladder, liver.
Gas (flatulence)	Sigmoid flexure, stomach, intestines.
General nervousness	Solar plexus, 7th cervical, coccyx, adrenals, back and shoulder muscles.
Glaucoma	Eyes, kidneys, coccyx, lymphatics.
Hay fever	Adrenals, ileo-cecal valve, intestines, stomach, liver, lungs, thymus.
Headache (general)	Genito-urinary tract, head, neck, eyes, spine, liver, stomach, large intestine.
Headache (migraine)	As above. Add 7th cervical, liver, coccyx.
Headache (top)	As above. Add gonads.
Headache (temples)	As above. Add eyes.
Headache (back)	As above. Add 7th cervical, solar plexus.
Headache (front)	As above. Add sinuses, ileo-cecal valve, 7th cervical, eliminative organs, *LUNG – KIDNEY – SKIN – BOWEL*.
Heart disease	Heart, 7th cervical, liver, stomach, intestines, gall bladder, spleen, solar plexus, kidneys, pituitary, thyroid, sigmoid flexure, shoulder girdle, adrenals.
Hemorrhoids	Edge of heel, liver, pelvic area, large intestine, spine, prostate, back of legs, either side of achilles tendon.
Hiatus hernia	Diaphragm, hiatus hernia reflex, stomach, work top of left foot between the tendons of 1st and 2nd toes toward the ankle, also back of left hand between the thumb and index finger
Hiccups	Solar plexus, diaphragm.
High blood pressure	Spleen, diaphragm, kidneys, large intestine, 7th cervical, coccyx, solar plexus.
High cholesterol	Liver, thyroid.
Insomnia	Inside of big toe, pituitary, or, press fingertips together for 10-15 minutes, or, solar plexus, 7th cervical and coccyx.
Jaundice	Liver, gall bladder.
Kidney stones	Kidney, ureter tubes, bladder, parathyroids, skin, lung, large intestine.
Leg aches	Coccyx, sciatic, hip, parathyroids, adrenals, low back.
Leukemia	Spleen, all lymph glands, thymus.
Lumbago	Kidneys, low back, spine, parathyroids, adrenals.
Migraine	See headaches. Add 7th cervical, coccyx, liver.
Muscle tone	Adrenal, pineal, pituitary, parathyroids.
Neck ache	Head, side of head, neck, 7th cervical, spine, shoulder, back muscles, whiplash reflex.
Nervousness	Solar plexus, solar plexus breathing 7th cervical, coccyx.
Prolapsed rectum	Sigmoid flexure, coccyx, back of leg near achilles tendon, prostate, large intestine, parathyroids, adrenals, pituitary, low back, spine.
Prostate	Prostate, sigmoid flexure, large intestine, spine, rectum, kidney, ureter tube, bladder, pituitary, neck, low back.

Sciatica	Inner side of ankle, sciatic reflex, colon, prostate, hip, buttocks, low back, sacrum, coccyx, shoulder, neck, jaw.
Sinusitis	Sinuses, thymus, lymphatics, head, eustachian tube, neck, ileo-cecal valve, stomach, pancreas, adrenals, small and large intestines.
Skin problems	Skin, kidney, lung, large intestine, adrenals, pancreas, sex glands.
Stiff neck	Shoulders, neck, 7th cervical, head, spine, shoulder joint.
Thyroid	Pituitary, thyroid, adrenals, sex glands, neck, shoulders.
Tonsils	Tonsil reflex, neck, lymphatics, large intestine, eustachian tube, solar plexus, 7th cervical.
Toothache	Teeth reflex, 7th cervical.
Tumors	Pituitary, pancreas, thymus.
Ulcers	Solar plexus, hiatus hernia and pylorus reflexes, diaphragm, stomach, small intestine, adrenals, 7th cervical, coccyx.
Varicose veins	Large intestine, liver, hip, buttock, low back, pancreas.
Whiplash	Milk big toe, work the neck, 7th cervical, shoulders, back muscles, cervicals, thoracic spine, solar plexus, 7th cervical, coccyx.
Women's problems	Pituitary, thyroid, adrenals, sex glands, fallopian tube, lymphatics in groin.

Questions to Discomforts and their major reflexes.

A person catches cold easily. What reflexes would you work on?

_____

Name 3 reflexes you would work for arthritis.

_____

When would you work the solar plexus? (Name at least 4)

_____

_____

What reflexes would you work for migraine heachaches?

_____

When there is back pain what reflex(es) other than the spine should you check? _____

Where there is hip trouble also check the: spleen_____ gall bladder_____ shoulder_____ spine_____ parathyroid_____ pituitary_____. (Check appropriate reflexes.)

Callouses on the feet sometimes serve a purpose. What might it (they) be? _____

When there are eye problems, work the reflexes to the: gall bladder_____ kidney_____ intestine_____ coccyx_____ neck_____.

Sinus trouble alerts you to work the respiratory system really well. TRUE_____ FALSE_____.

A person is extremely tired in the morning, improving as the day goes on, and, suffers from allergies. Which reflex would you concentrate on? Pituitary gland_____ kidney_____ adrenal gland_____ stomach_____ pancreas_____ gall bladder_____ spleen_____ intestine_____ 7th cervical_____ solar plexus_____.

Chapter 18
EXTRAS, TRICKS OF THE TRADE

Make sure that your hands are warm when you first touch the feet...the first touch is often the most important contact, since you are acquainting each other with the "feel" of hand on foot.

Rub, squeeze, stretch and shake your hands, to promote circulation. Limber up fingers and hands, and start the flow of healing energy that often exudes heat far greater than that of your natural body heat.

Become aware of the "energy zone" that you pass through, as you reach to touch the feet. Analyse the feeling as you approach and enter this field. Explore the foot with eyes closed, in order to contact your feelings, your intuition and your sensitivity. Explore the differences between the tendons of the foot; notice how it relates to back tension. Feel for temperature differences. Notice how different desserts affect different people in different ways. Learn about unique sensitivities of your own individual fingers.

Notice the resiliency of the foot...does it feel healthy? Does it indicate tension, degeneration? Does the foot feel hollow, with recessed areas, no resiliency...that may indicate poor nutrition, energy blockage, poor circulation.

AS YOU TOUCH, SO ARE YOU TOUCHED.

There is an energy exchange between your client and yourself. Give the best of yourself and you will receive tenfold what you give away.

A large portion of the brain affects the thumb and hand. As you work, with your hand touching the foot, it predisposes the activation of *your* spinal energy, activating the brain on many levels.

ALWAYS WASH YOUR HANDS AFTER A REFLEXOLOGY SESSION, to avoid the spread of infection, to clear any less than desirable energy that you may have picked up from your client, and, to announce to your client that her session is terminated...and that indeed, her feet are done!

Tips, herbs, points and positions other than Reflexology

Acne, cold sores, pimples
Use unpasteurized honey, which is analgesic, antibiotic, and has healing properties. Use it as if it were a lotion.

Antibiotics
Water and gardencress, garlic, horseradish, cranberry juice, nasturtium (all parts - in salad or as a tea).

Arthritis
Use devil's claw root, epsom salt baths (2 cups per tubfull) stay in the tub for 35 minutes, at least twice per week; extra calcium, 10 cherries and 5 almonds per day.

Bed sores
Coat with white sugar or honey for quick healing.

Bedwetting
Happens to bright active children, who have no time to use the "loo". New habits need to be installed. Daily, chew on a cinnamon stick, eat a piece of celery, drink 6 oz. of cranberry juice (this deals with odour). Go "spend a penny" *every* hour of the day. (Enlist the aid of teachers during school days, to facilitate the job.) *Allow* the drinking of water after supper to dilute fluids

in the bladder and avoid bladder irritation. Every evening, at bedtime, hold the bedwetting reflex (1st joint, palmar surface, of the pinky) for 60 seconds. Ten days of remaining dry constitutes a *cure*.

Bee stings
Rub with papaya or meat tenderizer which contains papain, or with a papaya tablet.

Body odour
Use chlorophyll tablets or pearles, add zinc to diet.

Bug bites
Rub bite with raw potato, relieves itch.

Burns
Immediately apply unpasteurised honey, removes pain, heat of the burn, and begins the healing process, is antibiotic. Honey cuts off the nitrogen from the air which causes the pain, and eliminates scarring if done immediately. May eliminate blisters. The most effective ointment for burns. Aloe, cider vinegar or vitamin E are also effective but honey seems to work best.

Cankers
Flush the mouth with yeast or acidophilous bacteria. Hold it in the mouth and swish it around.

Circulation
Dry brush massage, daily, before bathing. Add cayenne to the diet.

Colds
Immediately use Vitamin C, in fairly large doses, as much cranberry juice as comfortable, eat onion or garlic. Use Vitamin A for mucous and for the defence system, and take hourly doses of zinc gluconate. Eliminate dairy products until the cold is gone.

Cold feet
Put cayenne in your shoes. (Capsicum)

Cold (shivering)
Add cayenne (Capsicum) to the diet or take Capsicum tablets.

Colic
With your nails, gently scratch the back of the infant's hands, toward the wrist, using the back of your nails: weak fennel tea.

Constipation
Herbal bowel cleansers, not laxatives, walnuts in diet, capsicum, linseeds, psyllium seeds, some bran and fiber foods.

Convulsion
Step on or bite the pinky finger at the first joint to inhibit the seizure (especially effective in epilepsy).

Cramps (abdominal)
Both hands are placed alongside the centre line of the back of the head, press deeply, add calcium to diet.

Cramps (menstrual)
As above and press in on inner side of leg, 4 fingers above the ankle bone near the bone, but toward the back of the leg. Calcium and Dang Quei in diet.

Cramps (muscles)
Brush the cramped muscle gently, lightly with fingers. Do not clutch the cramped muscle. In a serious cramp pinch the area by the base of the nose, above the lip, where the skin and mucous membrane join. Hold it tightly until the cramp subsides. It is the same idea as a twitch on a horse or a ring on a bull's nose, it is a point for immediate muscle release.
Also if you sleep on your stomach hang your feet over the edge of the bed and in any position. Do not tighten the covers over the feet. If it is a leg or foot cramp, flex the foot or stand on it. Learn not to extend the foot when you stretch. Stretch the arms and legs but *flex* the foot while you do. Add calcium, magnesium, and maganese to diet.

Deafness
Exert pressure with a metal comb to the fingertips on the same side as the deafness, then on opposite side.

Dyslexia

Walk a few paces, then read a few lines from a book. Notice your inflection, spacing, comprehension and ability to read. Now, hold your hand over your navel and with the other hand, rub the acupuncture spots called K27 just below the collarbone, on both sides of the sternum, in a slight depression. Switch hands and repeat, this time repeating the alphabet out loud as you rub, from A to Z while rolling your eyes in *all 4 directions.* Now march in place, swinging your arms to touch the opposite knee, in what is known as *cross-crawl,* about 15-20 times, keeping your eyes turned up to the left. Then march in place moving right arm and right leg up simultaneously, then left arm and leg up simultaneously in a *homolateral-crawl,* eyes down right. Then repeat *cross-crawl.* Now read the page again, noticing the changes in comprehension, ability to read, spacing and inflection. *Hurrah!* Very simple and very effective for all ages!

Ear pain

Tuck a wad of cotton in the space between the last tooth and the angle of the jaw, bite down hard, repeat several times during the day. Hook in behind the soft palate, and stretch it forward. An onion poultice behind the ear and warm castor oil or oil of almond sweet in the ear often reduces or eliminates inflammation and its pain.

Energy lift

Perform a *cross-crawl* (see dyslexia for description) then a *homolateral crawl,* then back to the *cross-crawl.* Or hold your hands so that the backs of the nail phalanges (that entire joint) press firmly against each other, for 10 seconds, release and enjoy a 4-hour energy pick-up. Or, tap the thymus spot on the sternum, below the clavicle or, rub the K27 spot on the sternum, below the clavicle, in a small depression on both sides of the sternum.

Eye pain

Squeeze the knuckles of the index finger, hard, (or of the second finger if the eyes are wide apart), pressing upper and lower surfaces simultaneously for 5 minutes at a time. Place a slice of cucumber or a used tea bag on the eye to relieve burning.

Feet

For tired, hot or swollen feet, bathe them in potato water, wrap them in a towel, sprinkled with roasted salt.

Food poisoning
Flu symptoms, nausea,
or vomitting

Add two or three heaping teaspoons of cinnamon to some water, stir and drink swiftly (before it congeals and becomes difficult to consume). This takes 20 minutes to work. Repeat if necessary after an hour if only partially effective. If no effect, get medical attention.

Gall stones
Gall bladder flush

Take 6 oz. of *fresh* lemon juice and 6 oz. of pure olive oil. Starting after dinner, take one ounce of each one (don't mix them), wait 15 minutes, then take another ounce of each one, and repeat until you have consumed all 6 oz. of each (1 hour and 15 minutes). In the morning, after a night's sleep, check your bowel movement for bluish-green gall stones of varying sizes and numbers. Some people cramp a bit in the morning, generally there will be an emotional lift if the flush was successful, and often, taste changes (less sugar desired, etc.). If the flush is done twice yearly, you need only take 3 oz. of oil and 3 oz. of lemon juice, after the first year.

Headache

Press in at the corner of the webbing between the thumb and index finger. Press in with the index of the opposite hand for best angle, toward the thumb bone as well as downwards. Also, use the teeth of a comb, into the top of the ball of the hand (where fingers attach) then closing your fingers, squeeze the comb down into the ball of the hand. Or, press in and up at the base of the skull, in the hollow to the outside of the muscles going into the skull. Hold for 7 seconds. Add fresh lemon to coffee and drink it. Sometimes a hot cloth around the neck and a cold cloth on the area in pain will eliminate a headache.

Heartburn

Four to five rolled oats, chewed for a while then swallowed. The oats should be uncooked.

Hiccups

Press in straight on the solar plexus reflex in the hand and hold.

High blood pressure

Sit in a chair, with the left ankle over the right knee. With the right hand, hold the ankle, from above, over the top of the ankle. With the left hand, go below the foot and hold the pinky toe side of the foot. Your position is right if your arms cross near the wrist. Now, breathe in deeply, placing your tongue to the roof of your mouth and breathe out placing your tongue behind your lower teeth. Do this for 1 minute. Then place your feet firmly on the floor, and all five finger tips of each hand together (fingertips only, not quite prayer position) and continue the same breathing technique as before. Do this for one minute. This will reduce blood pressure.

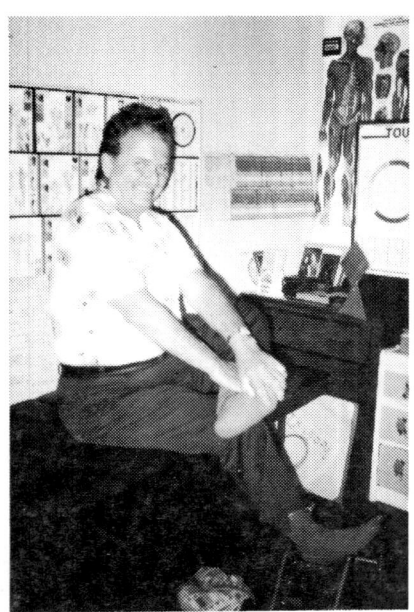

Insomnia

Work the inside of the thumb, and the inside of the big toe. Hold the spots to the side of the eyebrow (near the temples) and slightly above the eyebrow. Also contract first the feet, legs, thighs (one at a time) and so on up the body until every portion of you is tight. When every part of the body is tightened, hold that position for 20 seconds. Then let go all at once. Breathe in deeply 10 times to oxygenate the brain allowing you to fall asleep. Add calcium to the diet, some taken 1 hour before bedtime.

Legs tingly

Take Vitamin B6.

Lymphatics

One hand pushes firmly from the top of the ankle to the top of the thigh. As one hand finishes a sweep, the other has begun the same movement. Alternate swiftly. Can also be done from wrist to shoulder. Lumps and sensitivity denote need for lymphatic massage.

Memory

Add Gotu Kola, lecithin, and inositol to the diet. When trying to recall something, look up and generally to the left side of the brain.

Migraine

Use all headache remedies, and, also, place 1 or 2 drops of fresh lemon juice in nostril of the affected side.

Neck problems

Check teeth, dentures, jaw tension for possible TMJ problem. May require chiropractor or dentist for adjustment.

Nervousness

Clench the teeth and hands exaggeratedly for several minutes, then release.

Neuralgia	Press firmly against the upper palate in the mouth, just below the pain, or in the zone of pain, for 2 minutes. May need to be repeated for one week for total relief.
Pain	Place the tongue on the upper palate. Or, locate the spot beside the top of the coccyx or base of sacrum, on one side or the other of the body. You will find a little button that is quite sensitive. Hold that spot for 7 seconds. It is called the *cortisone button* and is an excellent pain relief technique. CAUTION: It does not remove the cause of the pain.
Pain (back of the body)	A metal comb in the palm with the teeth pressing into the fingers.
Pain (front of the body)	Bite down on the tongue will all your teeth for several minutes - it affects all ten zones.
Sciatica	With the opposite leg from the hurt one, while lying on your side on a bed, roll the opposite leg completely over the hurt leg and downward toward the floor. Check teeth, dentures.
Sedative	Stroke above the ear on the temporal lobe.
Senility (learning disabilities)	Breathe 12 times into a small paper bag, every half hour for 60 days in adult, 30 days for child, or, hold your breath every half hour. Causes opening of certain capillaries in brain and forces body to oxygenate. (see Dyslexia)
Sore throat	Gargle with acidophilous or yogurt. Onion poultice on neck.
Stomach ache	Pressure with the teeth of a comb to the first and second zones in the back of the hands. Run the comb, covering webbing between thumb and index. Run the comb or fingernails over the back of the hands for *nausea* or *motion sickness. Morning Sickness* - eat salted popcorn or raw oats.
Sunburn	Undiluted cider vinegar on entire burned area, takes out the sting, fever, burn, and may eliminate peeling.
Sweating hands	Press in straight on the solar plexus in the hand and hold.
Teething	Work the eye, ear and lung reflexes.
Tonifying the system	Place the person's hand on a lightly bent knee. The middle finger will be on the stomach 36 acupuncture point on the lateral side of the Tibia. Press this spot with your thumb, while the middle finger of your other hand presses along the outside of the leg on the calf, below the bone. Hold each point along the way for 5-10 seconds.
Ulcers	Drink 3-4 ounces of raw potato or raw cabbage juice (must be freshly made), 4-5 times per day. Water may be added, and you can mix and match the juices. It will heal an ulcer, but will only cure it permanently if you change your lifestyle. Cayenne (capsicum) will heal a bleeding ulcer.

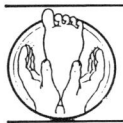

Chapter 19
PAIN, DIS-EASE, AND LOADED EMOTIONS

Pain is often like a fire alarm, asking you to *PAY ATTENTION* TO YOUR own system. Pain removal will be permanent if you also get to the root cause of the problem and eliminate it, or if the pain has become chronic. Pain causing tension, which tightens the muscles, squeezes nerves, alters circulation causing more pain, is chronic. Removing *ALL* pain from a sprained ankle, for instance, could be dangerous, since the person will then use or abuse it. Use pain control wisely. Leave a bit behind, as a reminder to the person to pay attention.

DIS-EASE is often the body's request for change. Change of job, of lifestyle, of nutrition, of emotions, or of attitudes. Help your friend to search for the change needed. Though patterns that are less than resourceful can often lead to certain illnesses. Following is a thought provoking list of some discomforts and the emotions associated with them:

Alcoholism	Inadequacy, poor self image, guilt, and pain too strong to cope with. Alcohol dulls the feelings.
Allergies	False pride or ego, over-sensitivity.
Arthritis	Squelched anger, bitterness, a person may feel unloved. Arthritics are most often gentle, sweet, giving, nurturing people, who might like to throttle somebody but wouldn't dream of it.
Asthma	Choking back of thoughts, words and emotions, over protection of self.
Back Problems	Insupportable load to carry. Lack of support in their lives, economic and emotional support is lacking.
Neck problems	Pain in the neck attitude. Inflexibility, refusing to see all sides of an idea. Stubborness about self and others. Pride.
Sciatic problems	Pain in the butt attitude.
Blood pressure	HIGH: Long standing, unresolved emotional problem. LOW: Defeatism, depression, sorrow.
Constipation	Holding onto old ideas, fear of change. Selfishness, stinginess, especially with regard to thoughts and emotions.
Deafness	Avoidance of others' communication. Too many internal voices (by voices I mean the voice that said "what voices? I don't have any voices!").
Diabetes	Little belief in life's sweetness. Deep sorrow. Emotional upheaval that may have caused it initially.
Diarrhea	Fear. Rejection of the past and present. Getting rid of ideas before they can be absorbed. Sometimes getting rid of old habit patterns before a change of lifestyle or attitude.
Fatigue	Resistance. Boredom. A need to change occupations or goals. Inability to "use" today, today.
Foot problems	Lack of understanding. Fear of taking a step in a new direction or forging ahead.
Gall stones	Bitter, hard thoughts.
Gout	Impatience. Anger. Domineering. Held in feelings of irritation.
Headaches	Tension. Emotional upset, hurt feelings, uncertainty, fear. In *Migraines,*

inability to cope with relaxation, or coming down from stress. Resistance to the flow of life, and sexual fears.

Heart Problems	Lack of joy, belief in pain, stress, pressure. Belief that the heart stores emotions rather than it just being a pump.
Hemorrhoids	Fear of letting go. Burdens, Pressure, tension.
Menopause problems	Fear of aging, loss of femininity. Fear of not being desirable or wanted.
Sinus problems	Irritation to particular people.
Shoulder problems	Problems too heavy to bear. Burdens. Work ethic attitudes.
Teeth problems	Indecisiveness, little ability to analyze.
Tumors	Nursed hurts and shocks.
Ulcers	Anxiety, dislike, discomfort, fear, tension with lifestyle, situation and job.
Varicose veins	Clogged ideas, discouragement.

These are a composite of common disorders. Of course, there are more emotional reasons for each. Take a good honest look at yourself, and make some new decisions, new goals. Remember – "If *it* doesn't work for you, *CHANGE it.*" Do it differently.

Take responsibility for your health and your choices and help others around you to do the same.

Chapter 20
ADDITIONAL REFLEXES

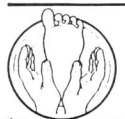

Bunions, gout, prostate, reproductive organs
Energy, inflammation (all the "itis's") for anything that ends in 'itis'
Kidney
Around ankle bone, systemic. Press from outside in towards the bone. Constipation, foot problems congestion, construction, energy.
Lymphatics
Outside ankle, ovary, testes, constipation, drainage from lymph intestines and lungs, hip bone, mucous
Neck
Balance Point
Neck/shoulder
Pituitary, Breathing
Sleep point
Eyes
Bladder, ureter stricture, cramps
Ear, cough, headache, insomnia.
Foot, hangover, indigestion, sinus, toothache
Flatulence, foot, forearm, hemorrhoids, shoulder joint, toothache
In front of ankle bone, constipation, cough, foot, vomitting
5th Lumbar
Sacrum
Liver
Coccyx
Breathing, spleen, pancreas

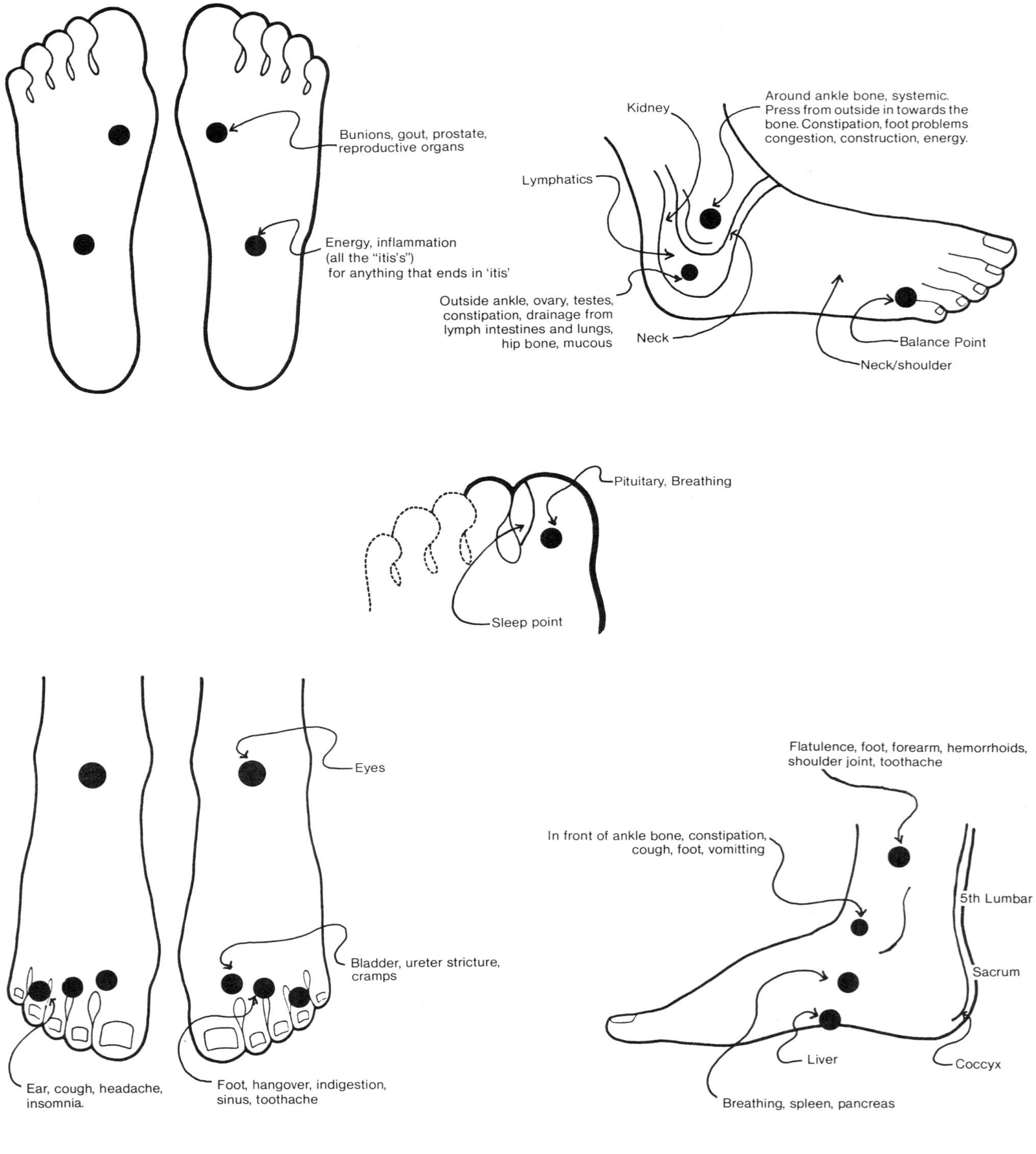

Fig. 23. Additional Foot Reflexes

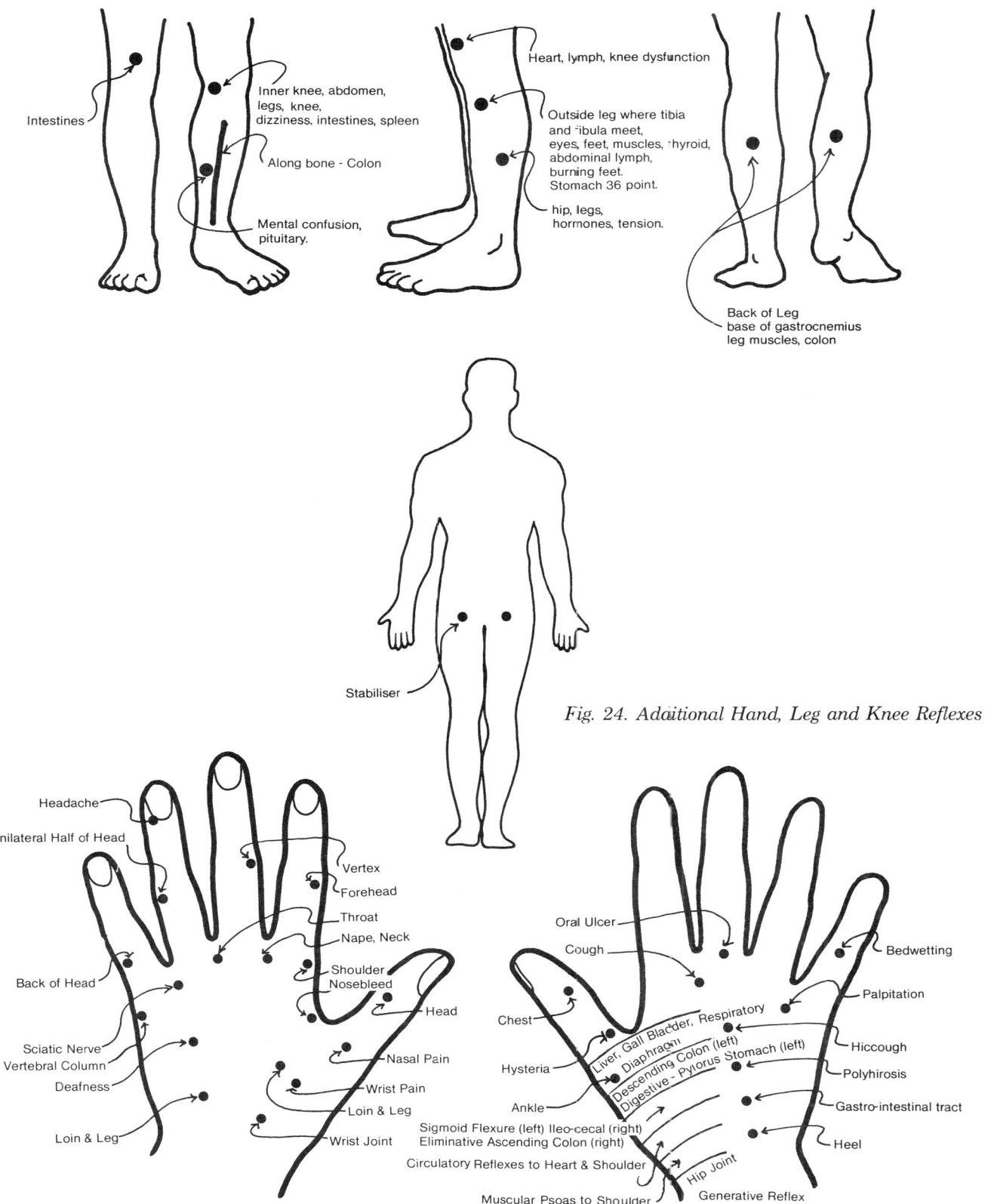

Intestines

Inner knee, abdomen, legs, knee, dizziness, intestines, spleen

Along bone - Colon

Mental confusion, pituitary.

Heart, lymph, knee dysfunction

Outside leg where tibia and fibula meet, eyes, feet, muscles, thyroid, abdominal lymph, burning feet. Stomach 36 point.

hip, legs, hormones, tension.

Back of Leg base of gastrocnemius leg muscles, colon

Stabiliser

Fig. 24. Additional Hand, Leg and Knee Reflexes

Headache

Unilateral Half of Head

Back of Head

Sciatic Nerve
Vertebral Column

Deafness

Loin & Leg

Vertex

Forehead

Throat

Nape, Neck

Shoulder
Nosebleed

Head

Nasal Pain

Wrist Pain

Loin & Leg

Wrist Joint

Oral Ulcer

Cough

Chest

Hysteria

Ankle

Liver, Gall Bladder, Respiratory
Diaphragm
Descending Colon (left)
Digestive - Pylorus Stomach (left)

Sigmoid Flexure (left) Ileo-cecal (right)
Eliminative Ascending Colon (right)

Circulatory Reflexes to Heart & Shoulder

Muscular Psoas to Shoulder

Hip Joint

Generative Reflex
Vital Force

Bedwetting

Palpitation

Hiccough

Polyhirosis

Gastro-intestinal tract

Heel

117

Areas where there is swelling, stiffness, discolouration, excess body hair, moles, spots, warts on the spots shown in this and the following page, may indicate weakness of the corresponding organ. This may also be true if the person is sensitive when pressure is applied to these spots.

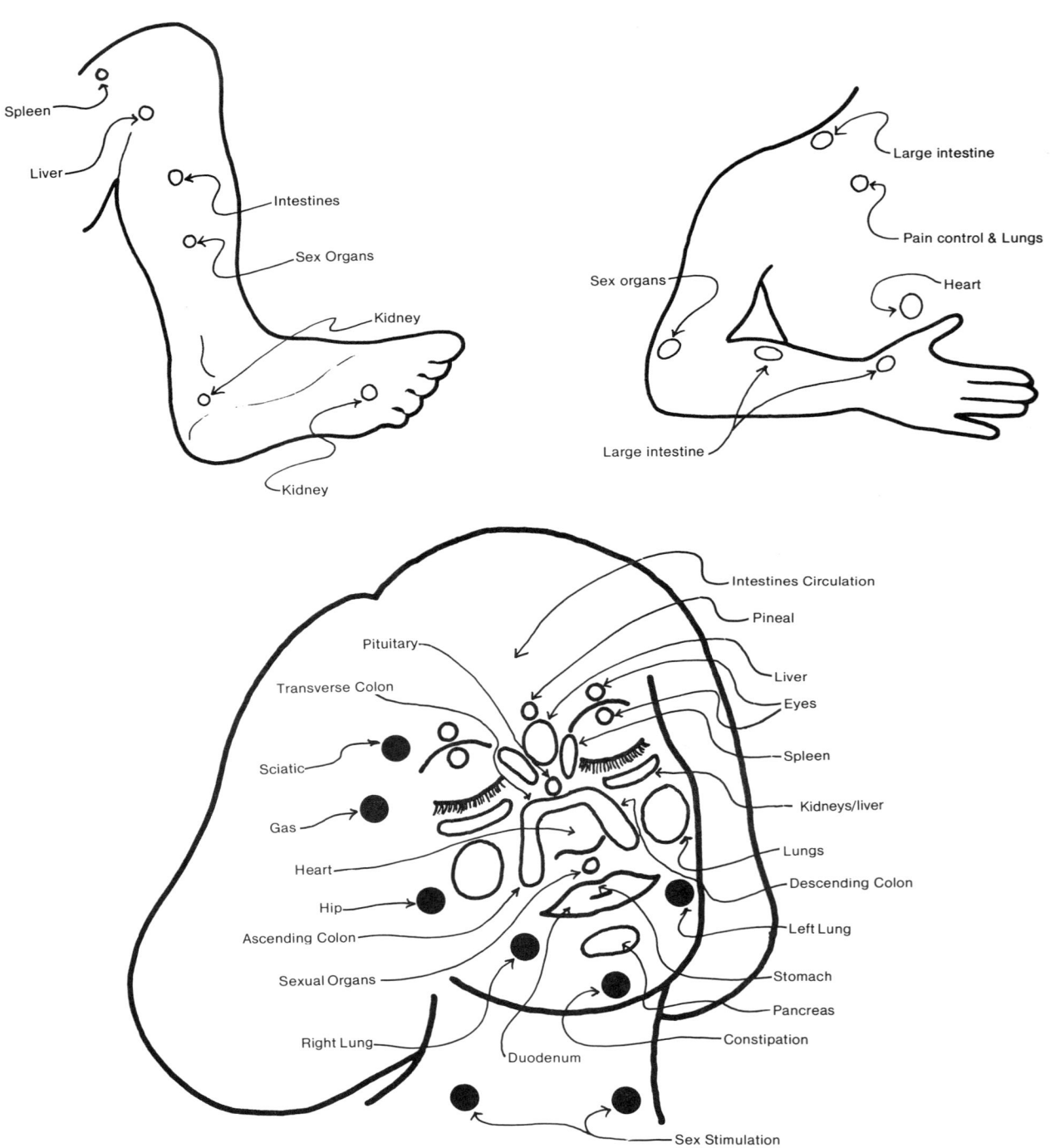

Fig. 25. Leg, Torso/Arm and Face Reflexes

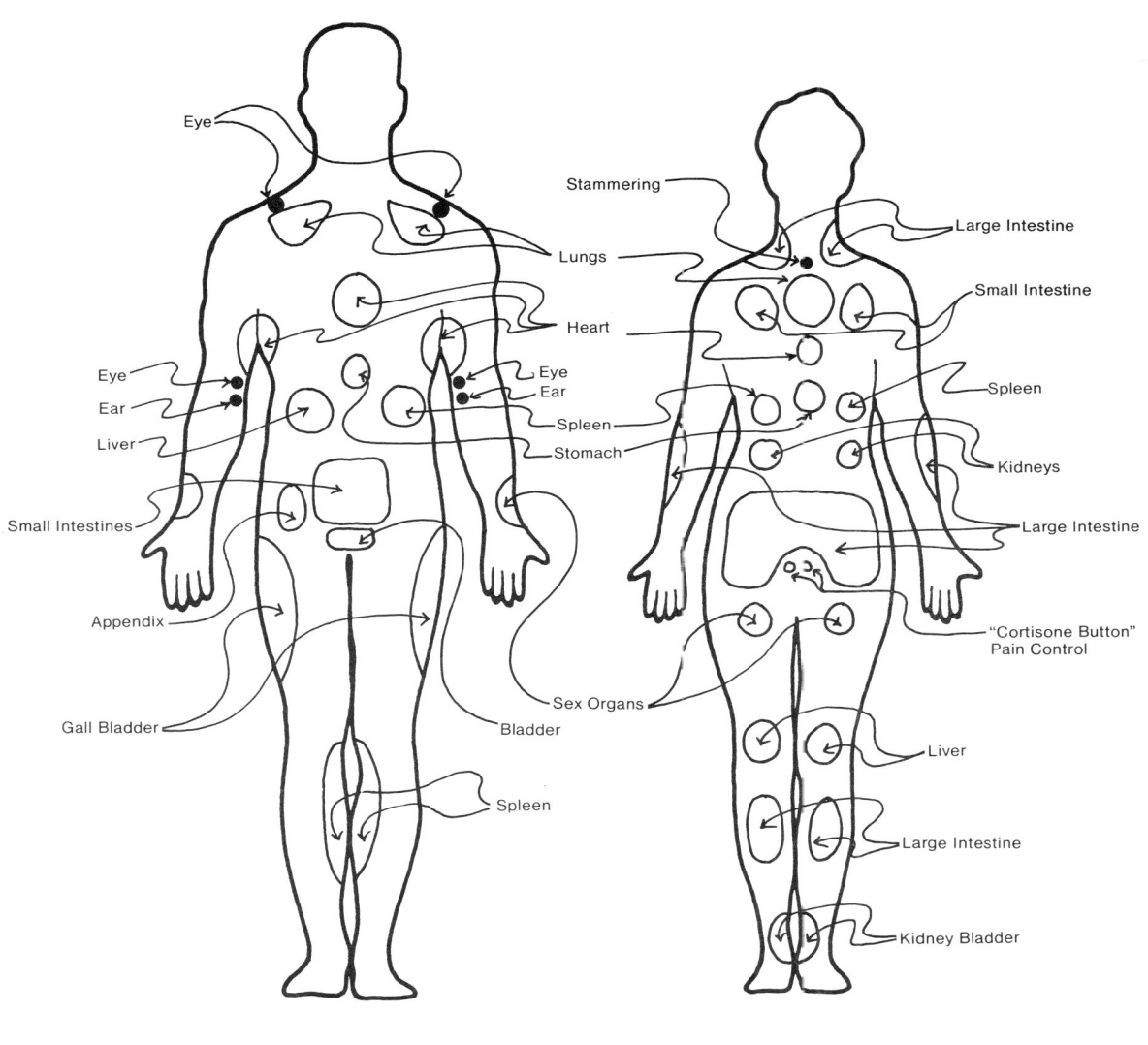

Body Reflexes - Frontal　　　**Body Reflexes - Back**

Fig. 26. Body Reflexes

Chakras

Each chakra draws in its own special vital energy from the physical atmosphere. It is discharged along the nervous system, flowing through the fatty sheaths not their fibres and is distributed throughout the body. Surplus and devitalized particles are released through the skin and breath. This exchange is vital to health. Use this information as you see fit.

People cover or emphasize the chakra they are most involved with.

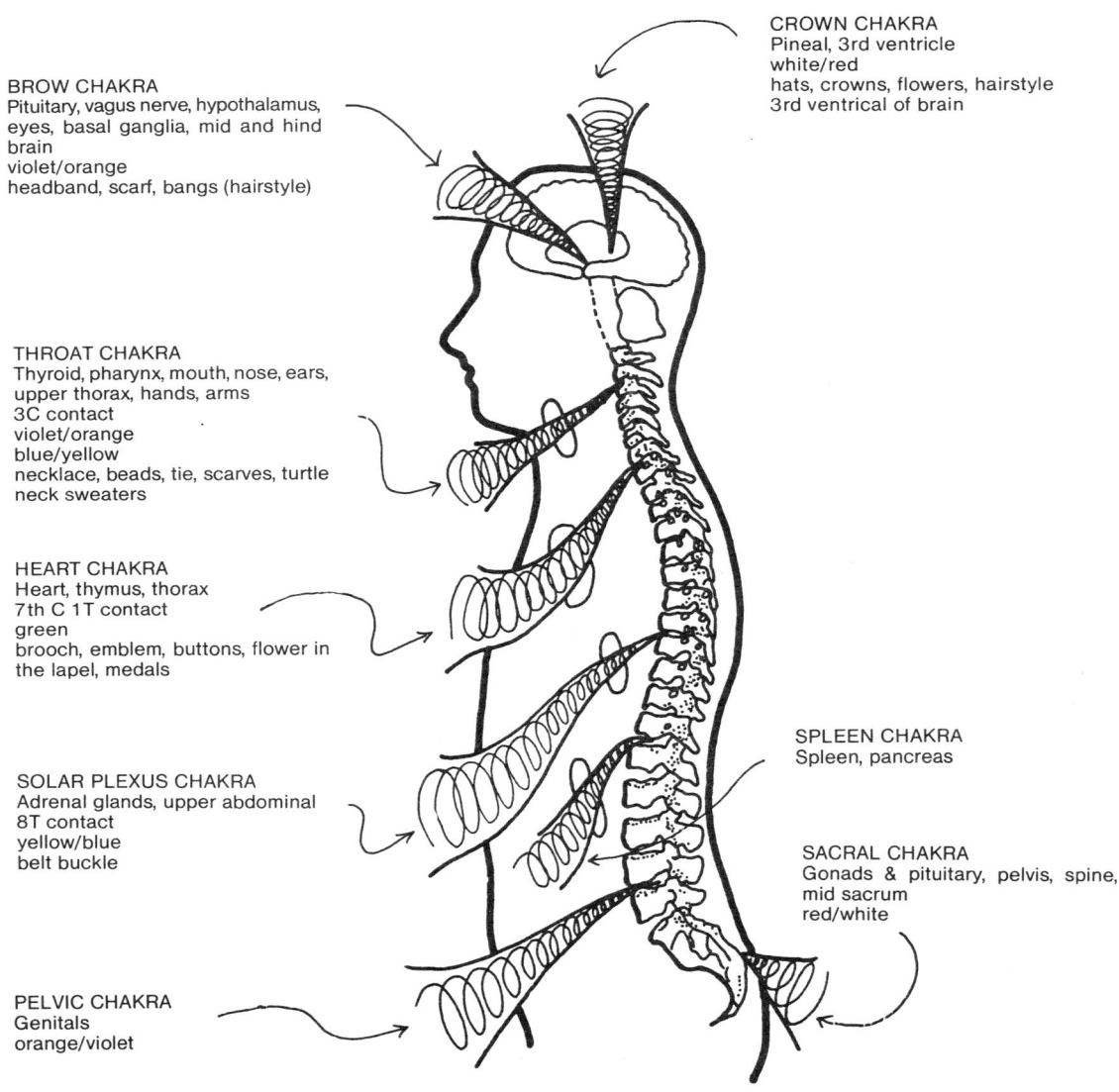

CROWN CHAKRA
Pineal, 3rd ventricle
white/red
hats, crowns, flowers, hairstyle
3rd ventrical of brain

BROW CHAKRA
Pituitary, vagus nerve, hypothalamus, eyes, basal ganglia, mid and hind brain
violet/orange
headband, scarf, bangs (hairstyle)

THROAT CHAKRA
Thyroid, pharynx, mouth, nose, ears, upper thorax, hands, arms
3C contact
violet/orange
blue/yellow
necklace, beads, tie, scarves, turtle neck sweaters

HEART CHAKRA
Heart, thymus, thorax
7th C 1T contact
green
brooch, emblem, buttons, flower in the lapel, medals

SPLEEN CHAKRA
Spleen, pancreas

SOLAR PLEXUS CHAKRA
Adrenal glands, upper abdominal
8T contact
yellow/blue
belt buckle

SACRAL CHAKRA
Gonads & pituitary, pelvis, spine, mid sacrum
red/white

PELVIC CHAKRA
Genitals
orange/violet

Fig. 27. The Chakras.

The Polarity Experience Simplified

Holding positive, negative and neutral poles relaxes a person, helping the energy flow, and feels good. Use polarity when it seems suitable.

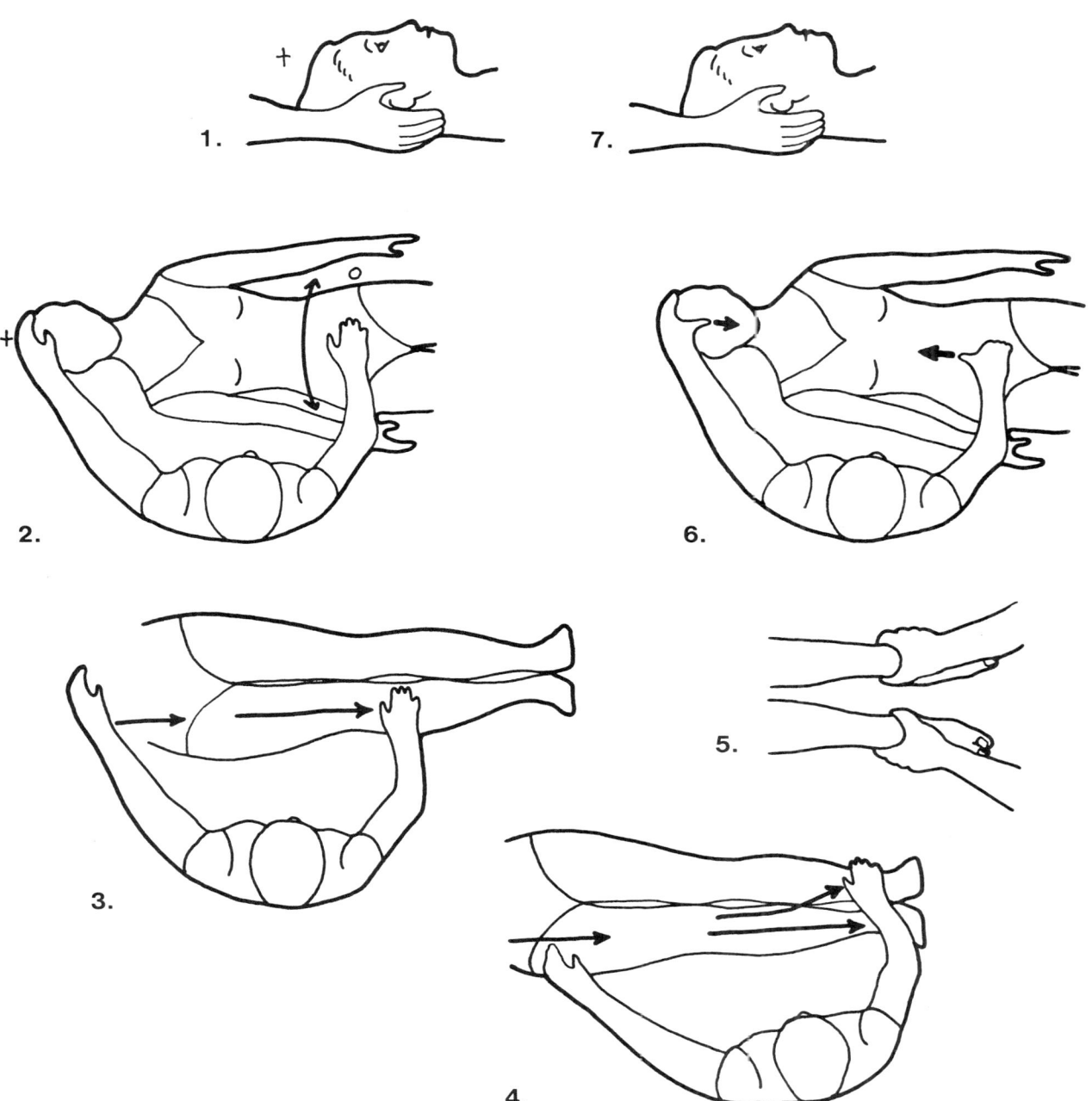

Fig. 28. The Polarity Experience.

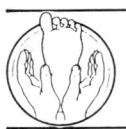

Chapter 21
SOME MANIPULATIONS OF THE FOOT AND TOES

Sometimes a person needs just a bit more on the foot than reflexology. Perhaps the foot hurts if the arch is not quite correct, causing discomfort. There are instances where small manipulations are helpful. All of them affect portions of the body as well as the foot itself.

For low arch

On the right foot, place the left hand so that it cups the heel, with the thumb on the ankle bone and its third phalange on the cuboid bone, on the lateral side of the foot. The right hand goes under the medial arch, with the thumb over the top of the foot.

Now perform a quick twist with the right hand and a short, quick thrust with the left hand.

This will loosen the big toe joint, reposition the cuboid bone, raising the arch.

It also reflects to the mid-body and tonifies the system. Most people say that it feels good.

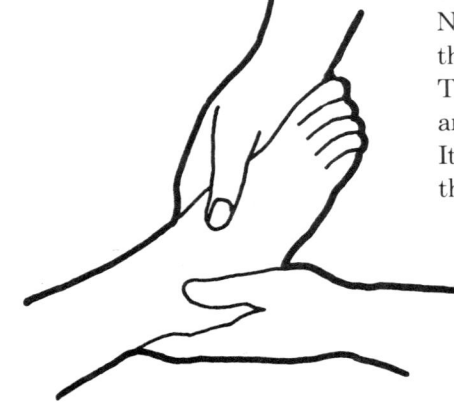

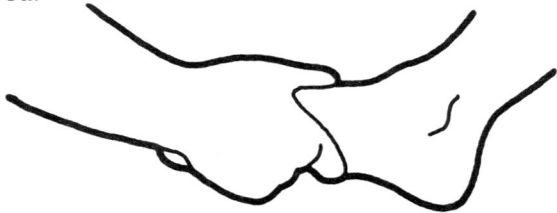

Fig. 29a). Some Manipulations for Low Arch

For high arch

On the right foot, the right hand lies over the top of the foot. The middle finger rests firmly on the highest point on the top of the arch. The thumb is on the ball of the foot, across the lung reflex. The left hand covers the right hand with its middle finger over the same contact point. The thumbs cross on the ball of the foot.

Now push the foot toward the person, middle fingers pushing against the contact spot, then a quick, short pull toward yourself rearranges the foot, often audibly.

This manipulation affects the mid-back.

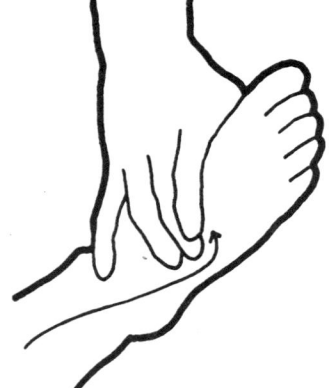

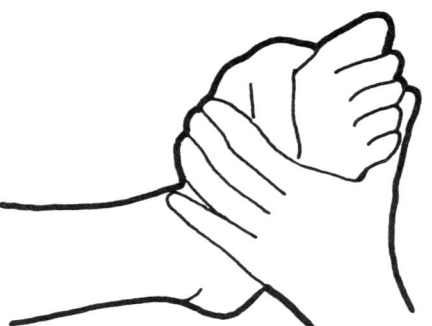

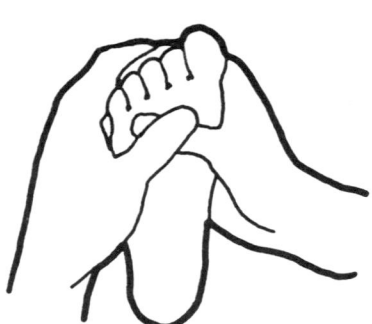

Fig. 29b). Some Manipulations for High Arch

Big toe adjustment

Stand to the person's right, facing the foot. the right hand goes over the toes, with the fingers on the ball of the foot and the thumb over the big toe. Quickly thrust the toes downward, while pushing the arch up.

This affects a tension release in the shoulders and respiratory tract.

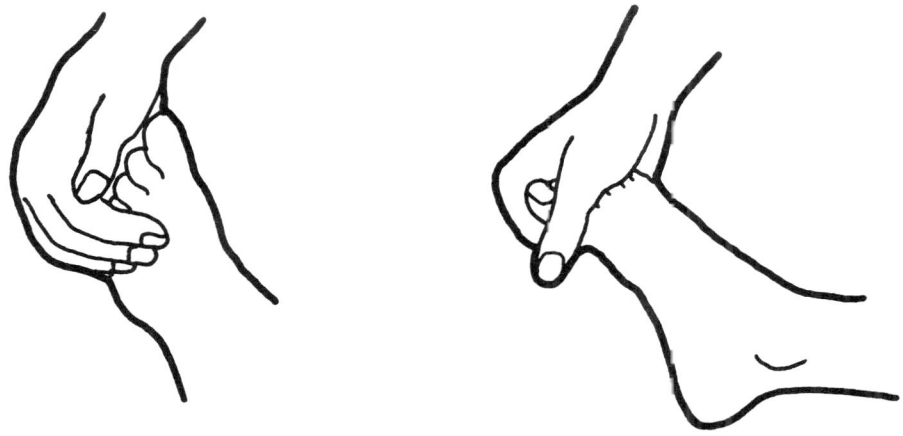

Fig. 29c). Some Manipulations for Big Toe Adjustment

Bunion and big toe adjustment

On the right foot, the left thumb holds the dorsal portion of the big toe, while the fingers anchor the ball of the foot.

With the pad below the thumb of the right hand, smack the bunion smartly and sharply. This will release the lock and fixation of the bones and cartilage. Even a light tap may prove painful if there is a fixation, and may turn blue where venous stasis is released.

If the big toe is sore to begin with, just pull up on the big toe and the other toes.

It is an excellent manipulation for bunions that also affects neck problems, shoulder tension, sciatica, prostate and uterine problems.

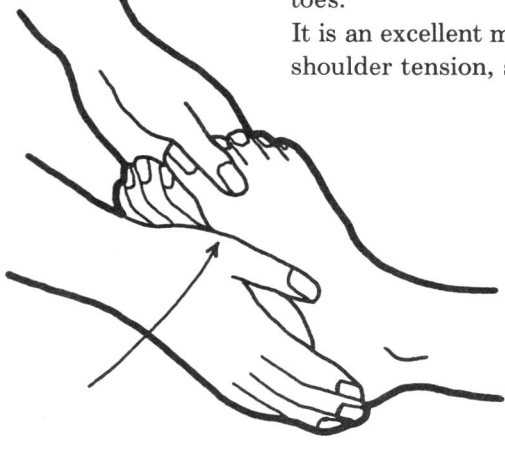

Fig. 29d). Some Manipulations for Bunion and Big Toe Adjustment

Gait   Sometimes a person's gait may not be synchronized; when he walks, one leg takes a longer stride than the other. This may explain why a person walks in a circle when lost in the woods since, with each longer stride, he may veer to one side.

This imbalance may come from a muscular difference in the legs, from over-tiredness, from emotional stress affecting the legs or from faulty messages received from both hemispheres of the brain.

The correction is actually based on acupuncture meridians. Work the spots shown quite firmly. They will be sensitive, even a bit painful.

Explain to your friend that these spots are uncomfortable so that he is prepared, since the sensation is different from the usual reflexology spots. The points are located at the tops of the joining toes on both feet. There is no spot between third and fourth toes.

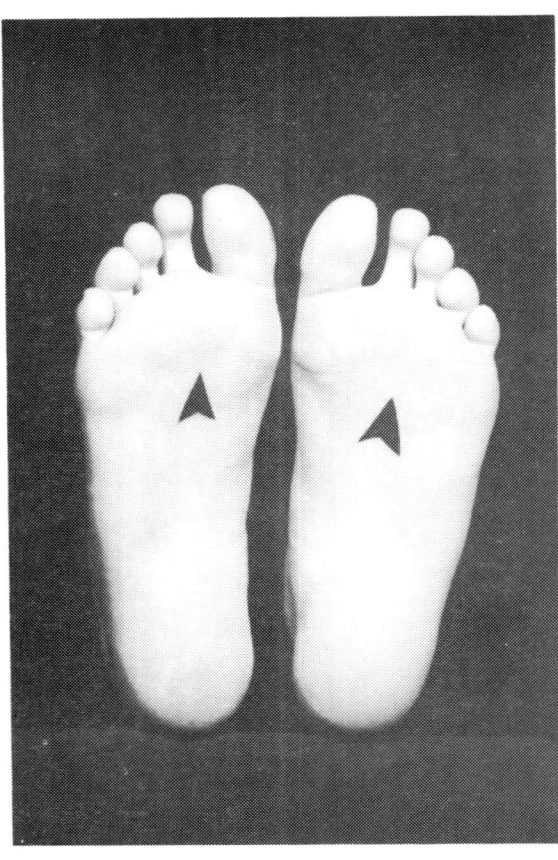
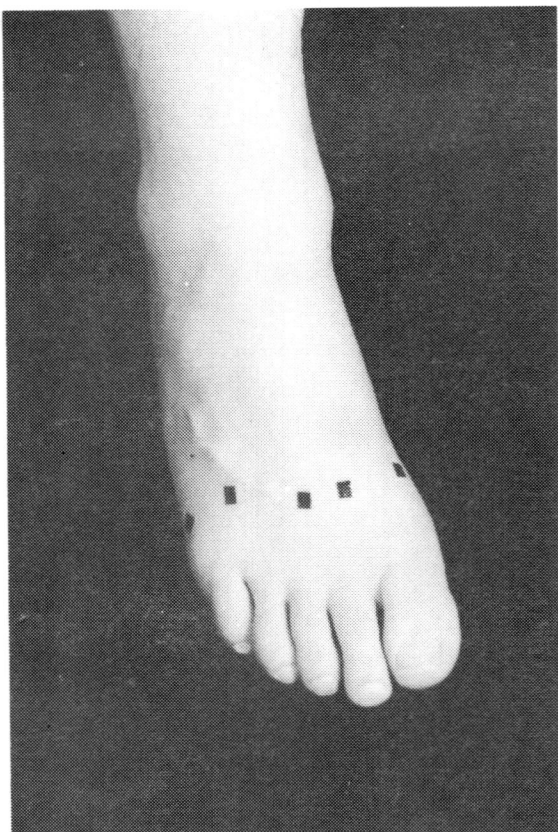

Dis-abilities of the Foot

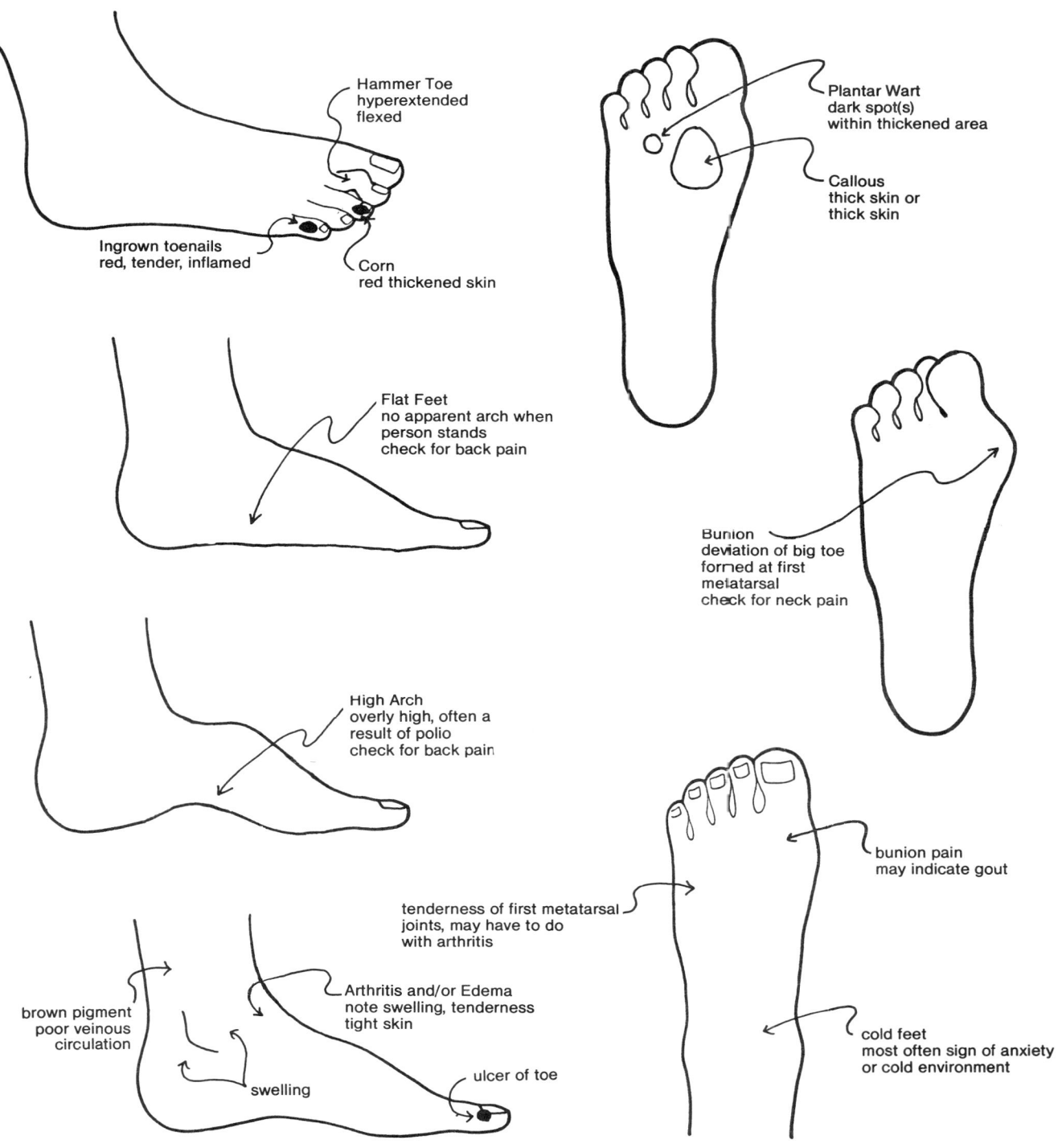

Fig. 30. Dis-abilities of the Foot

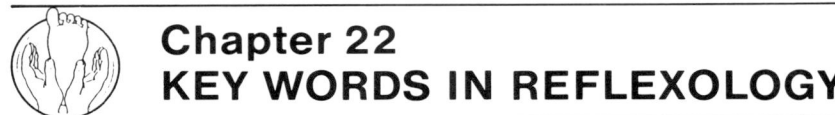

Chapter 22
KEY WORDS IN REFLEXOLOGY

FUNCTION	AREAS INVOLVED	WHAT YOU WORK
Relaxation	Nerves, hormone balance.	Work reflexes to: solar plexus, 7th cervical, coccyx, pituitary, pineal, thyroid, parathyroid, adrenal, sex glands, thymus.
Circulation	Blood, lymph, nerve supply.	Spleen, liver, heart, lymph, head, spine.
Assimilation	Stomach, and small intestine.	Stomach, small intestine, gall bladder, pancreas.
Elimination	Large intestine, kidney, lung, skin.	Large intestine, kidney, lung, skin.

Chapter 23
STAYING LEGAL

It is illegal to treat and/or diagnose anyone in any way, whether paid or not, except as a licensed physician.

It is illegal to tell someone to stop doing something that a doctor has told them to do.

It is illegal to identify or imply disease or health problems through Reflexology.

It is illegal to say that any food, substance or technique will cure a condition or problem.

It is illegal to say you will try to help.

It is **NOT** OK to cause pain.

It is **NOT** OK to cause fear.

It is **NOT** OK to cause someone to depend on you totally for their well being.

It is OK to say "hmmmm".

It is OK to show someone something about their posture, their reflexes.

It is OK to help someone determine their own imbalances.

It is OK to teach someone the reflexes that might change their body's response, and they can let you teach them.

It is OK to talk about the importance of food, exercise, touch and supplements without being specific.

It is OK to say you might be able to relieve discomfort.

It is OK to look up things in your notes when you have doubts.

It is OK to say you've worked with others and *THEY* have had success.

It is OK to ask your friend if your pressure is comfortable or if something is sensitive.

It is OK to talk or play music or be silent.

It is OK to make mistakes.

Reflexology complements conventional medicine and other alternate techniques. It does not replace them.

Chapter 24
VITAMINS, MINERALS, HERBS – HOW TO USE THEM

Their uses and where to find them

When and How to take vitamins

Vitamins are best absorbed when they are taken with other foods and minerals since they are a food. The best time is after meals and as evenly throughout the day as is possible. If they must be taken all at one time, the best results will be obtained if they are taken after the largest meal, after dinner rather than breakfast. Since Vitamin C aids in the absorption of iron, they should be taken together. Calcium aids the absorption of Vitamin D and zinc aids in the absorption of Vitamin A. So it's best to take Vitamins and Minerals together. Vitamin E, however, may affect iron adversely in the intestinal tract, so, if you can, take Vitamin E ten or twelve hours before or after minerals containing iron. But remember it is best to space various vitamins throughout the day if you are able to.

Celery stalks

Celery stalks contain potassium, sodium, calcium, phosphorous and iron. It is excellent for nerves and the leaves contain Vitamins A, B and C. Celery juice can help to ward off arthritis, relieve heartburn and can be a very good antidote for alcohol.

Other vegetables

Turnips have Vitamin A, B and C. Peppers have Vitamin P. Green beans are great for kidneys, heart and rheumatism. Spinach is rich in iron, but don't eat it if your liver gets upset. Eggplant is good for bowels. Cucumber (peel and all) eliminates water from cellular tissues, dissolves uric acid.

Cereals

Cereals – millet – are high in protein. Remember that wheat and milk are allergy offenders and mucous producing.

Eliminate from diet

Eliminate totally from your diet: white bread, white sugar refined, pasteurized *coloured* butter and margarine. Watch for additives and preservatives.

Herbs

Herbs have many healing qualities and can be used as teas, in tablet form, as poultices and even as hand and foot baths. Each herb has specific qualities. In combination, herbs of differing effects are combined to work on a systemic approach, to equalize and revitalize the body. A general combination would contain one part passive or soothing to an injury, (demulcent) one part nourishing, strengthening, and aromatic, and one part eliminative (causing perspiration, urination, defecation). In general add 1 teaspoon of herb to a cup of boiling water, cover and let steep for five to seven minutes. Another generalized rule is to take an herb for ten to twenty days, then stop for ten to twenty days, then resume for another ten to twenty days.

V I T A M I N S

SR=Supplementary Ranges T=Toxicity	● Function ○ Deficiency symptoms	Natural Sources	● Best taken with. ○ Depleting factors
A SR 10,000 - 25,000 I.U. T 50,000 I.U.	● body tissue repair and maintenance, resisting infection, night vision, kidney repair and maintenance, skin, eyes, bones, teeth, blood protein digestion, liver. ○ burning eyes, night blindness, skin blemishes and dryness, fatigue, infections, loss of smell, slow growth, bleeding gums.	Dark green and yellow fruit and vegetables, fish liver oil, liver, apricots (dried), spinach, parsley, carrots, eggs, canteloupe, tomato.	● B Complex, C, D, E, and F, Choline, Calcium, Zinc, Phosphorous. ○ alcohol, caffeine, cortisone, excess iron, mineral oil, vitamin D deficiency, tobacco.
B1 Thiamine SR 2 - 50 mg T unknown	● appetite, learning, blood building, carbohydrate metabolism, circulation, digestion, hydrochloric acid producing energy, muscle tone, intestines, stomach, heart, nervous system. ○ nervousness, irritability, numb hands and feet, short breath, poor appetite, depression, fatigue, sensitivity to noise.	Molasses, brown rice, fish, meat, poultry, nuts, brewer's yeast, wheat germ, brazil nuts, sunflower seeds, organ meats, whole grains, legumes.	● B Complex, extra B6, C, Phosphorous, E, Manganese, Sulpur. ○ alcohol, caffeine, fever, raw clams, excessive sugar, stress, surgery, tobacco.
B2 Riboflavin SR 2 - 50 mg T unknown	● antibody and red blood cell formation, cell respiration, metabolism of carbohydrates, fat, protein. ○ cataracts, sores and cracks in corner of mouth, itchy burning eyes, red sore tongue, stress, dizziness, digestive problems, nervous instability.	Molasses, nuts, organ meats, whole grains, nuts, avocado, peach, dark green vegetables, red hot pepper, rice bran, egg yolk, sesame, sunflower, chestnut, legumes.	● B Complex, extra B6, C, Phospherous. ○ alcohol, caffeine, excessive sugar, tobacco.

	Functions / Deficiency	Food Sources	Supplements / Depleted by
B3 **Niacin** SR 30 - 50 mg T over 50	● circulation, growth, hydrochloric acid production, metabolism of carbohydrates, sex hormone production, digestive system, adrenals, nervous system, skin, hair, teeth. ○ fatigue, depression, headaches.	Brewer's yeast, seafood, lean meats, milk products, poultry, disiccated liver, whole grains, rice bran, prunes, apricots, peaches, citrus, nuts, kelp, hot red pepper, mushrooms, fish, green vegetables.	● B Complex, extra B1, B2, C, Phosphorous. ○ alcohol, antibiotics, caffeine, corn, excessive carbohydrates, stress, sugar. NOTE: diabetics who take niacin should do so with care.
B6 SR 4 - 50 mg T unknown	● antibody formation, digestion, hydrocholoric acid production, fat and protein utilisation, weight control, maintenance of sodium/potassium balance (nerves). ○ acne, anemia, arthritis, high cholesterol, hair loss, atherosclerosis, baldness, inflammation of mouth, bursitis.	Soy beans, liver, salmon, bananas, oranges, wheat, bran, beef, cod, sunflower seeds, molasses, brewer's yeast, prunes, brown rice, peas, green leafy vegetables, beets, lemon, corn and peanut oils.	● B Complex, extra B1, B2, Pantothenic Acid, C, Magnesium, Potassium, Linoleic Acid, Sodium. ○ alcohol, birth control pills, caffeine, radiation, x-rays, tobacco.
B12 SR 5 - 50 mg T unknown	● blood cell formation and cell longevity, healthy nervous system. ○ allergies, anemia, arthritis, bronchial asthma, bursitis, epilepsy, fatigue, low blood sugar, insomnia, over weight, shingles, stress, speech difficulty.	Cheese, fish, milk products, organ meats, eggs, tuna.	● B Complex, Choline Inositol, C, Potassium, Sodium. ○ alcohol, caffeine, laxatives, tobacco.
Choline SR 100 - 1,000 mg T unknown	● lecithin formation, liver and gall bladder regulation, nerve transmission, metabolism and transport of fat and cholesterol, hair, thymus, kidneys. ○ high cholesterol, constipation, dizziness, ear noises, headaches, heart palpitations, high blood pressure, low blood sugar, insomnia, bleeding stomach ulcers, hypertension.	Eggs, liver, brewer's yeast, fish, legumes, peanuts, soy beans, lecithin, wheat germ, brain.	● A, B Complex, B12, Folic Acid, Inositol, Linoleic Acid. ○ alcohol, caffeine, excessive sugar, insecticide.
Folic Acid SR 1,000 - 10,000 mcg T unknown	● hydrochloric acid production, protein metabolism, red blood, reproduction, growth, liver. ○ anemia, alcoholism, atherosclerosis,	Green vegetables, milk, organ meats, oysters, salmon, whole grain, dates, roots, brewer's yeast, oysters.	● B Complex, B12, Choline, Linolenic Acid. ○ stress, caffeine, alcohol, tobacco, streptomycin.

baldness, diarrhea, fatigue, menstrual problems, mental illness, stomach ulcers, stress.

Inositol
SR 100 - 1,000 mg
T unknown

● fat and cholesterol metabolism, bone marrow, eye membranes, hair, vital organs.
○ hardening of arteries, cholesterol reduction, stipation, eczema, eye abnormality, hair loss, baldness, heart disease, overweight.

Molasses, citrus fruit, brewer's yeast, meat, milk, nuts, vegetables, whole grains, lecithin, soy beans.

● B Complex, B12, Choline, Linoleic Acid.
○ alcohol, caffeine.

Pantothenic Acid
SR 20 - 100 mg
T unknown

● antibody formation, carbohydrate, fat, protein metabolism, skin, adrenals, use of riboflavin, growth.
○ allergies, fatigue, arthritis, diabetes, baldness, cystitis, digestive disorders, premature aging, low blood sugar, kidney trouble, tooth decay, stress.

Brewer's yeast, legumes, organ meats, salmon, wheat germ, whole grains, liver, fresh orange juice, egg yolk, mushrooms, salmon.

PABA (para-anime acid)
SR 10 - 100 mcg
T toxic for some if taken frequently.

● production of folic acid, skin, hair, intestines, sunscreen, utilization of proteins.
○ constipation, depression, digestive disorders, fatigue, irritability, graying hair, over-active thyroid, rheumatism, sunburn, lack of pigment.

Molasses, brewer's yeast, liver, organ meats, wheat germ, green vegetables.

● B Complex, Folic Acid, C.
○ alcohol, caffeine, sulfa drugs.

B15 Pangamic Acid
SR 100 mg
T unknown

● glands, heart, kidneys, nerves, muscles, energy, cell oxidation and respiration, metabolism, glandular and nervous system stimulation.

Brewer's yeast, brown rice, rare meats, seeds, organ meats, whole grains.

● B Complex, C, and E.
○ alcohol, caffeine.

C
SR 250 - 5000 mg
T above 5000 mg for some if taken regularly.

● adrenals, infection resistance, iron assimilation, blood capillary walls, connective tissue, skin, ligaments, gums, heart, teeth.
○ allergies, colds, infections, athero-

Cabbage, papaya, strawberries, broccoli, oranges, peppers, potatoes, citrus fruits, fresh fruits and vegetables.

● Rutin hesperidin, Biflavinoids, all Vitamins, Minerals. With colds: Vitamin A and Zinc Gluconate.
○ antibiotics, aspirin, high fever, stress, tobacco, mercury, cortisone, air

	Functions / Uses	Food Sources	Helpers / Destroyers
(continued)	sclerosis, arthritis, baldness, high cholesterol, low blood sugar, heart disease, hepatitis, insect bites, overweight, prickly heat, sinusitis, tooth decay, scurvy, bleeding, anemia, shortness of breath, bursitis, bruising, gout.		pollution, DDT, excess water.
D SR 500 - 1500 I.U. T 25,000 I.U. Toxic to some if taken regularly	● skin, bones, heart, nerves, teeth, thyroid gland, blood clotting, skin respiration, calcium absorption. ○ alcoholism, allergies, cystitis, eczema, psoriasis, stress, bone disease, teeth and gum problems, rickets, retention of phosphorus in kidney, colds.	Egg yolks, organ meats, bone meal, sunlight, salmon, tuna, herring.	● Vitamin A, C and F, Choline, Calcium, Phosphorous. ○ mineral oil.
E SR 50 - 600 - 1200 dependent upon the need T over 4,000 for some if taken regularly	● internal: anti-clotting, male potency, lung protection, muscle and nerve maintenance, hemoglobin maintenance, heart. ● external: capillaries, skin, hair, cell respiration. ○ internal: allergies, arthritis, atherosclerosis, baldness, high cholesterol, cystitis, diabetes, heart disease, heart problems, menstrual problems, menopause, migraine, overweight, phlebitis, sinusitis, thrombosis, enlarged prostate, impotence, varicose veins, aging, retardation. ○ external: burns, scars, warts, wrinkles, wounds.	Dark green vegetables, eggs, liver, organ meats, wheat germ, vegetable oils, dessicated liver, peanuts, whole grains, soybeans.	● Vitamin A, B Complex, B1, C, F, Manganese, Selenium, Phosphorous. ○ birth control pills, chlorine, mineral oil, rancid fat and oil, air pollution, inorganic iron.
F SR 10% of total calories T unknown	● blood pressure, glandular activity, growth, lubrication, sex organs, skin, hair, cell structure, calcium availability. ○ allergies, baldness, bronchial asthma, heart disease, high cholesterol, gall bladder problems or removal,	Vegetable oil, wheat germ, sunflower seeds, cod liver oil.	● Vitamin A, C, D, and E, Phosphorous. ○ radiation, X-rays.

eczema, leg ulcers, psoriasis, rheumatoid arthritis, overweight, underweight.

	Uses / Symptoms	Sources	Related
K SR 300 - 500 mcg T unknown	● preparing women for childbirth, bile absorption, liver, longevity, blood coagulation. ○ bruising, eye hemorrhage, gall stones, hemorrhaging, menstrual problems.	Molasses, yogurt, green leafy vegetables, sunflower oil, kelp, alfalfa, milk, cauliflower, fish liver oil, polyunsaturated oils.	○ aspirin, antibiotics, mineral oil, radiation, X-rays, rancid fat and oil.
P **Bioflavonoids** SR 500 - 3,000 mg T unknown	● bones, ligaments, gums, teeth, blood vessel walls, flu and cold prevention. ○ asthma, bleeding gums, colds, eczema, dizziness (inner ear), hemorrhoids, high blood pressure, miscarriage, rheumatic fever, bruising skin.	Fruit (skin, rind and pulp), apricots, cherries, grapes, grapefruit, lemons, plums, paprika, blackcurrants, tomato, parsley, onion, garlic, citrus.	● Vitamin C, Rutin. ○ same as Vitamin C.
Rutin **(a biflavinoid)** SR 50 - 100 mg T unknown	● vascular system, vessel integrity. ○ hemorrhoids, constipation, varicose veins, bruising.	Citrus rind, buckwheat.	● Vitamin C, Biflavinoids. ○ same as Vitamin C.

M I N E R A L S

	Uses / Symptoms	Sources	Related
Calcium SR 1,000 - 2,000 mg T for some if taken regularly.	● bone and tooth formation, heart rhythm, nerve tranquiliser, muscle growth, blood clotting, use of iron. ○ muscle cramps, sleeplessness, tooth decay, arm and leg numbness.	Milk products, molasses, bone meal, papaya, dark green vegetables (except spinach, beet green, rhubarb, chard), shell fish, nuts, seaweeds.	● Vitamin A, C, D, and F, Iron, Magnesium, Manganese, Phosphorous. ○ stress, lack of exercise, hydrochloric acid.
Chromium SR 100 -300 mcg T unknown	● blood sugar level, glucose metabolism, energy. ○ atherosclerosis, glucose intolerence, hypoglycemia, diabetes, retarded growth.	Brewer's yeast, cloves, corn oil, whole grains, cereals, clams, meat, liver.	○ air pollution.

Copper
SR 2 - 4 mg
T 40 mg

● bone formation, hair and skin colour, healing processes of the body, hemoglobin and red blood cell formation.
○ general weakness, impaired respiration, skin sores, anemia, retarded growth.

Beans, alfalfa, nuts, organ meats, seafood, raisins, molasses, bone meal, green leafy vegetables, seaweeds, soybeans, whole grains, fish.

● Cobalt, Iron,, Zinc.
○ excessive Zinc.

Iodine
SR 100 - 1,000 mcg
T unknown

● energy production, metabolism, thyroid, physical and mental development, hair, skin, nails, teeth, speech, mentality.
○ excess fat, cold hands and feet, irritability, nervousness, obesity, dry hair.

Seafood, kelp, iodized salt, seaweeds, fish liver oil, mushrooms.

Iron
SR 15 - 50 mg
T 100 mg or excessive dose for some.

● growth, protein metabolism, myoglobin, bones, brain, muscles, hemoglobin production, stress and disease resistance.
○ alcoholism, anemia, colitis, menstrual problems, breathing difficulties, brittle nails, fatigue.

Molasses, figs, raisins, fish, meat, poultry, dessicated liver, green vegetables, dried fruits, seaweeds, nuts.

● Vitamin B12, C, Folic Acid, Calcium, Cobalt, Copper, Phosphorous.
○ caffeine, excess phosphorous, tea, excess zinc, bleeding, diarrhea.

Magnesium
SR 300 - 500 mg
T 30,000 mg for some.

● acid/alkaline balance, blood sugar metabolism (energy), nerves, absorption of calcium, and Vitamin C, bones, enamel, arteries, heart, memory, glands, muscles.
○ nervousness, pain in upper half of body (ear infection, neuralgia), confusion, easily aroused anger, rapid pulse, tremors, soft bones, kidney stones, tooth decay.

Bran, honey, green vegetables, nuts, seafood, spinach, comfrey, bone meal, kelp, dolomite.

● Vitamin B6, C, and D, Calcium, Phosphorous.
○ alcohol, diuretics, high cholesterol.

Manganese
SR 1 - 50 mg
T excessive doses for some.

● enzyme activity, reproduction, growth, sex hormone production, Vitamin E utilization, important to

Bananas, bran, celery, cereals, egg yolk, green leafy vegetables, legumes, liver, nuts, pineapple, whole grains,

○ excessive calcium, phosphorous.

carrot, beet, buckwheat.

pituitary gland, muscle coordination.

○ ear noises, dizziness, loss of hearing, paralysis, convulsions, glandular dissorders.

Phosphorous
SR 800 - 1000 mg
T unknown

● bone/teeth formation, cell growth and repair, energy production, heart muscle contraction, kidney function, metabolism of calcium and sugar, nerve and muscle activity, vitamin utilisation.

○ irregular breathing, nervous disorders, over-weight, weight loss, bone disease and weakness, gum and teeth disease.

Eggs, fish, grains, yellow cheeses, seeds, green vegetables, seaweeds, legumes.

● Vitamin A, D, and F, Calcium, Iron, Manganese.

○ excessive aluminum, iron, and magnesium, sugar, antacids.

Potassium
SR 100 -300 mg
T unknown

● heartbeat, muscle contraction, nerve tranquilisation, fluid balance, protein and glucose absorption, growth.

○ acne, continuous thirst, dry skin, fatigue, general weakness, insomnia, muscle damage, poor reflexes, high blood pressure, nervous.

Dates, figs, peaches, tomato juice, sunflower seeds, molasses, raisins, dried apricots, bananas, potato, fish, whole grains, green vegetables.

● Vitamin B6, Sodium.

○ alcohol, caffeine, cortisone, diuretics, laxatives, excessive salt and sugar, stress.

Selenium
SR unknown
T unknown

● increases effectiveness of Vitamin E to oxygenate blood, cancer preventative, protects against radiation, cadmium, mercury, prevents chromasome damage, reduces cholesterol, helps synthesise protein.

○ high blood pressure, insomnia, premature aging, inflexibility, arteriosclerosis.

Brewer's yeast, garlic, liver, eggs, brown rice, tuna, broccoli, cabbage, tomatoes, onions, mushrooms.

○ mercury poisoning.

Sodium
SR 100 - 300 mg
T 14,000 mg for some

● cell fluid level, proper muscle contraction, blood, lymph system, nerves.

○ appetite loss, excess symptoms –

Salt, milk, cheese, seafood, meats, poultry, green vegetables, chard, kale, celery, seaweeds, soft water.

● Vitamin D, Potassium.

○ lack of chlorine and lack of potassium, excessive perspiration.

Sulphur
SR trace
T unknown

thirst, shrinkage, edema, high blood pressure.

● body tissue formation, nails, nerves, hair, skin, elimination, liver.
○ flatulence, brittle nails and hair.

Bran, cheese, clams, eggs, nuts, fish, wheat germ, cabbage, kale, brussel sprouts.

● Vitamin B Complex, B1, Biotin, Pantothenic Acid.

Zinc
SR 20 - 100 mg
T unknown

● burn and wound healing, carbohydrate digestion, prostate gland function, reproductive organ growth and development, sex organ growth and maturity, Vitamin B1, Phosphorous and protein metabolism.
○ loss of taste, poor appetite, poor wound healing, retarded growth, fatigue, stress, hyperactivity, slow healing, prostatitis, sterility, baldness.

Brewer's yeast, liver, seafood, spinach, sunflower seeds, mushrooms, paprika, whole grains, maple syrup, leafy vegetables, soybeans, bran.

● Vitamin A, Calcium, Copper, Phosphorous.
○ alcohol, excessive Calcium, lack of Phosphorous.

Alfalfa	For pituitary gland, arthritis, chlorophyll, highly nutritive, alkalizes body rapidly, detoxifies body, and liver.
Aloe vera gel	For burns, scratches, bites, bed sores, acne and other skin irritations.
Aloe vera juice	Digestion, ulcers, milk laxative, general tonic.
Bee pollen	Increase energy and stamina, improves digestion by aiding in assimilation, asthma, allergies and prostate disorders.
Black cohosh	Female estrogen, menstrual cramps, high blood pressure, poisonous bites.
Black walnut	Rids the body of parasites and tape worms.
Capsicum	Catalyst for all herbs, stops external and internal bleeding, circulation, use for nerves with lobelia, healing, stimulant, heals ulcers.
Chamomile	Nerves, toothache, helps stop smoking, alchohol, muscle pain.
Chaparral	Cleaner, arthritis, blood purifier, acne, boils.
Chickweed	Bronchial cleaner, eats carbohydrates (fat), deafness, pertonitis.
Comfrey root	Blood cleaner, ulcers, stomach, kidney, bowel, aids muscle and bone healing, aids lungs.
Damiana	Sexual impotency, reproductive organs, overcomes, loss of nerve, energy to limbs.
Dandelion root	Blood purifier, skin disorders, eczema, psoriasis, cramps, constipation, asthma, arthritis, aging, good in treating diseases of the liver, high in Vitamin A.
Dang Quei	Female problems, menstrual cramps.
Eyebright	Aids vision, the uppermost parts of the throat as far as the windpipe.
Garlic	Digestion, hypertension, equaliser of blood circulation, improves the physical condition of the body, works well in killing harmful bacteria.
Ginger	Stimulates circulation (pelvic area), gas, indigestion, paralysis of tongue.
Ginseng	Male hormone, longevity, prostate. stomach problems.
Golden seal root	Antibiotic. Acts like insulin. Cleanser, morning sickness, cure-all type of herb, pyorrhea, internal bleeding.
Gotu Kola	Mental troubles, blood pressure, energy, depression, longevity, strengthens heart, memory and brain, nervous breakdown.
Hawthorne berry	Aids nutritional deficiencies related to cardiovascular system. Best if used with capsicum.
Kelp	Thyroid, arteries, nails, hair falling out, cleanses radiation from body.
Licorice root	Natural cortisone, hypoglycemia, adrenal glands, stress, voice, colds.
Lobelia	Strong nerve relaxant, emetic in large amounts, asthma, angina pectoris, epilepsy, strengthens muscle action, weak heart, use with capsicum.
Mullein	Pain killer, respiratory organs, pulmonary complaints, excellent nervous soporific.
Poke root	Aids in relieving kidney and liver congestion, aids in breaking down mucous inside the intestine and sinus system, helps expel waste.
Safflowers	Natural hydrochloric acid (utilizes sugar of fruits and oils), skin disease, neutralizes uric acid, gout, hypo and hyperglycemia.
Sarsaparilla	Male hormone, rheumatism, gout, psoriasis, antidote for poison.
Thyme	Suppressed menstruation, nerves, colic, gas.
Uva ursi	Diabetes, kidneys, hemorrhoids, spleen, liver, pancreas.

Valerian root	Nervous disorder, nervous headache, pimples, muscle twitching, spasms, measles, fever, hysteria, promotes sleep.
White oak bark	Use in douches and enemas, varicose veins, loose teeth, bladder, goiter, gallstones, kidney stones, fever, bathe scabs, sores.
Wood betony	Indigestion, stomach, cramps, worms, jaundice, Parkinson's Disease.
Yellow dock	Blood purifier, cleaner, acne, high in iron, runny ears, tones entire system.
Yucca	Blood purifier, beneficial for arthritis and rheumatism.

Just like most other plants on this earth, herbs seem to work better when combined with similar acting herbs. When you have several herbs in combination, this relieves one of the possibilities of error in judgement which is inherent in the use of a single herb.

Gastrointestinal	Comfrey leaf, cayenne, pepper, myrrh gum, peppermint.	Gastritis, heartburn, indigestion, colitis, diverticulitis, ulcers, and over-eating.
General cleansing	Garlic, chaparral, red sage, mandrake, quassia, foenugreek, black cohosh, golden seal.	Degenerative disease, headaches, allergies, overweight, high blood pressure, chronic infections.
Respiratory	Slippery elm, foenugreek, thyme, pleurisy root, lobelia, Yerba Santa.	Bronchitis, mucous and phlegm accumulation, chronic cough, pleurisy, asthma.
Female irregularity	Red raspberry, damiana, crampbark, licorice, squaw vine, sarsaparilla, black cohosh, ginseng.	Amenorrhea, dysmenorrhea, cramps, discharge, menopause. Helps depression, low estrogen. Balances hormones, stimulates brain.
Nervous disorders	Valerian, hops flowers, lady slipper, lobelia, chamomile, scullcap, mistletoe.	Restlessness, insomnia, hyper irritability, hysteria, depression, worry, nervous headaches, relaxes.
Fluid irregularity	Alfalfa, parsley, buchu, uva ursi, corn silk, juniper.	Burning on urination, difficult urination; edema, frequency of urination.
Vermifuge-parasites	Garlic, black walnut, quassia, mandrake.	Used for 10 days, stop for 10 days, repeat for 10 days, stop for another 10 days and repeat for 10 days.
Sugar levels	Chaparral, ginger, blueberry leaves, dandelion root, golden seal, bilberry leaves, walnut leaves.	Diabetes, antibiotic, helps metabolism, may help eliminate or reduce insulin needs.
Temperature	Blue vervain, comfrey, buckthorn bark, yarrow, chamomile, cinchona bark, yarrow flowers.	Brings down fever, causes hormones to activate. Fever comes out in a sweat. Taken hourly until fever reduces - reduce and continue for 3-4 days.
Flu	Yarrow, chamomile, pleurisy root, blessed thistle, catnip, hyssop.	Thwarts neausea and vomiting, dries up diarrhea. Needs to be taken hourly for 8 hours.

Male irregularity	Cayenne, marshmallow, golden seal, ginger, juniper berry.	Prostate problems, reduces swelling, natural sedative. Stimulates circulation.
Appetite depressant	Poke root, chickweed, fennel.	Take this half an hour before meals.
Muscle	Hawthorne berry, cayenne, valerian, peppermint, passion flower.	Stimulates muscle of heart. Regulates heart beat, normalizes heart. Palpitations. Causes calm, increases circulation.
Loose elimination	Comfrey, pepsin, wheat germ.	Colon, pancreas. Reduces mucous in colon. Bad to have loose elimination because you lose too many enzymes, vitamins and minerals.

This formula is a herbal and digestive combination, which was popularized by Dr. William D. Kelly, who used it to dissolve the mucous film which coats the small intestine in many individuals. When this occurs, nutrients cannot get through the intestinal wall properly and therefore are not absorbed into the blood stream.

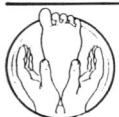

Chapter 25
SOME EFFECTS OF COLOUR

I mentioned in a previous chapter that I use colour during my sessions. Here are some of the ways in which I might use those colours:

Red Invigorates, stimulates the system. For anaemia, poor blood circulation, coldness, poor iron and minerals, for the liver and heart. Not for very emotional people or where there is pain. It allows energy and dynamic self to emerge as mental tensions ease.

Pink Affects pelvic problems, hip and buttock problems. Loving feelings. Not to be used on a bed in cases of insomnia.

Orange Stimulates and warms emotions and glands. Expands the emotional self, allows mental confusion to lift, self focus to sharpen, courage to increase, hearing to be more discerning. Stimulates the bowels, respiratory tract, milk production, relieves gas and sluggish bowel. Improves the assimilation of calcium, decreases menstrual cramps. It's good to use in thyroid problems. Not a good colour for weight loss.

Yellow Clear thinking and self expression, happiness. Relieves mental tension, integrates parts of the self. Stimulates the nervous system and brain activity and the appetite. Enhances liver and gall bladder function, dissolves arthritic deposits.

Lemon Loosens mucous, activates the thymus gland, builds bone, heals and eliminates the common cold, soothes muscular tension.

Green Relieves emotional stress and monetary caused stress. Practicality is stimulated. It balances the system neurologically, cleans the blood, calms the body/mind. Effective in high blood pressure, hot flushes, menopause, infection. Stimulates the pituitary.

Turquoise Aches and pains are reduced. Builds up the skin.

Blue Calming, soothing. Affects creative expression, encourages hope, perception discernment, quiets internal voices, balances body fluids, calms sleep, reduces fever. Stimulates the pineal gland.

Indigo Raises spirituality, awareness of strengths and self image. Physical co-ordination is heightened, protects the body from over-activity, balances metabolism and awareness of any imbalance. Sedative for pain and swelling, firms the skin.

Violet Stimulate intuitiveness, calms inner confusion, heightens introspection, reduces guilt and false pride, but rightful deserving is enjoyed. Provides insightful dreams, slows down motor functioning. Acts as an antibiotic and a builder of white corpuscles in the spleen. Depresses the appetite.

Purple Slows the heartbeat, reduces heart pain, increases venous drainage. Good for stiffness, congestion and excessive menstruation.

Scarlet Stimulates the heartbeat and arterial action, peps up kidney and adrenals.

White Assist all colours, heightens their positive value for each part of yourself.

I use coloured towels and *colour breathing* within a session. I send a *laser beam of blue* where there is acute pain. Colours sent and colours seen seem to affect the body. Often I will ask the person I'm working on to absorb certain colours and send them to specific areas in the body that I feel will benefit from that particular shade, or that particular colour.

Is it really being beamed? I don't know. Does it work? Absolutely! If you have a strategy that is beneficial, does it really matter if its it *true* or *real?* We make our own realities and each of our realities is *true* for the individual. If something works without any adverse effects – *USE IT!*

Our eyes often play with internal visuals – colours, shapes and symbols. They are there for our use, and our creativity.

Creative visualization also works. See yourself cleaning out your lung or your friend's, using scrub brushes, vacuum cleaners, cleansers, polishes, and whatever. Make the lung (kidney, colon etc...) look *pretty.* You need not know anatomy – a spine may appear to you as a linked group of spools of thread – with one of the spools off centre – well, push it in! A nervous system might look like Christmas tree lights with several bulbs blown. Imagine removing the old one, replacing it with a new one. Let the child in you play with symbols, colours, and your very own creativity. Then, watch for results, and let the child in you be filled with glee.

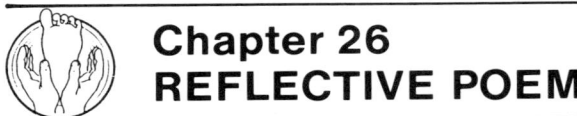

Chapter 26
REFLECTIVE POEM

The **pituitary** in the **big toe** will vary, centre it so it won't be contrary;
For muscles and memory to the **pineal**, on the side of the **big toe** near the **nail**.
The **neck,** oh, heck, at the **big toe's** base, with **thyroid, parathyroid, tonsils, vocal chords, 7th cervical** and **lymph** – a race for space.
The **head** reflex is in the **big toe**, if you don't use your **head**, you'll be a Schmo!
The **little toes** are the **head's** fine tuning for **sinuses** and tubes **eustachian.**
The **ball of the foot** sticks out as does the **chest,** with its **lungs, bronchial tube, thymus, heart** and **breast,**
and **diaphragm** and **solar plexus** below, they make you feel best.
With **eyes, ears** and **shoulders** at the **top of the ball,**
and **back muscles** on the **top** of the **foot** to make you stand tall.
In the **arch,** where they won't touch the ground,
the **liver** and **gall bladder** on **right** foot will be found,
with **stomach, pancreas** and **spleen** in same area on the **left**
and **adrenals** on both to give you a lift.
From **ileo-cecal** on the **right heel,** rise the **colon** then the **transverse**
across to the **left** foot, **descending** converse.
It sure is easy to remember this verse.
Angling to **sigmoid** and then to the **rectum,**
and **inside,** all mixed up is the **small intestine.**
Across the **ankles** from bone to bone, the **lymph** in the groin will tend to **roam.**
Below the **ankle** bones on the sides, **uterus** and **prostate** are on the **insides,**
while on the **outside** track the **ovaries** and **testes,** work them lightly and fairly "hasties"
The **spine** follows the **arch** from **toe** to **heel,** it often hurts so give it a fair deal,
then start again, but follow the **arch bone,** around the **ankle bone** and up the **heel.**
Under the **outside ankle bone** and around, **sciatic, hip, low back,** pain may abound.
Then just forward a bit, **hip, knee, low back** in the **soft triangle,** just in front of bony ankle.
The **bladder** is where there's a **puff** on the side of the heel, then alongside
the **tendon** for the **ureters** you'll steal,
cross the waist to find the **kidney,** well, my friends, are you still with me?
The foot is done, it feels great it feels fine,
Relaxation and a great big smile.

NOTE: There is a purpose for this poem! Sing it to a series of nursery rhyme tunes and you will remember all your major reflexes – or write a simple tune, send it to Touchpoint and we will publish it, tape it, and make it part of the Reflexology course.

Chapter 27
THE DAILY DOZEN

1. Keep your nails trim – neither too short nor too long. Wash your hands before and after every session.

2. Observe the foot for injuries, sprains, bruises, etc...

3. Work on a referred reflex if there is injury or damage (e.g. wrist for ankle).

4. Your only tools are gentle hands, fingers, and thumbs – no pencils, rods, not even knuckles; they may bruise or damage the feet.

5. No lotions, body oils, or bathing before a session. They make the foot slippery and hard to hold. reflexes will not be exact, energy exchange is hampered, and when bathed there is a *false* relaxation which will not give you a proper idea of the sensitivity of the foot. You can oil or bathe the feet at the end of a session, if you wish.

6. Avoid the words *treatment, patient, and cure*. We are not M.D.s. *Session, sitting, consultation, client, person, relieve stress or pain* – those are OK.

7. Results – sometimes they are immediate; most often, 4-8 weeks will elapse. Chronic problems – 2-3 visits per week (often, light and swift session). We work on the cause, not just the symptom.

8. Tell people of possible reaction – nausea, light headedness, dizziness. This is common and will pass quickly. Work the kidney well to help eliminate the toxins.

9. Maintain visual contact with your client; watch for signs of discomfort and back off when there is sensitivity.

10. Reflexology cannot harm – it can only normalize. Don't overwork, either in length or in strength.

11. Maintain high ethics, professionalism, concern and caring – especially with the medical field. We complement each other, we need each other. Never alter a client's medication or go against a physicians orders.

12. Above all – enjoy your work. Work is LOVE made visible.

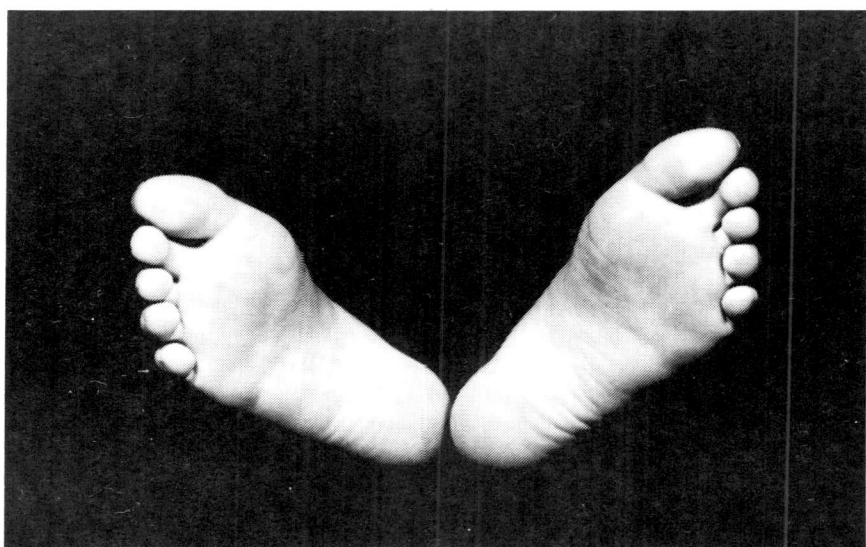

Chapter 28
A REFLEXOLOGY SESSION – STEP-BY-STEP

The following is a guide for a Reflexology sitting starting at the top of the foot, edging down the heel. Interspersed are various relaxation *desserts*. Once you feel comfortable with Reflexology, you'll find that your hand will wander to the area where they are most needed. Note that we alternate from plantar surface (sole) to dorsal surface (top) when we work to rest the thumbs while using fingers. The alternative sequence is described in this *session*.

A. Big toe

1. Pituitary
2. Hypothalamus
3. Pineal
4. 7th cervical
5. Neck
6. Thyroid
7. Parathyroid
8. Vocal chords
9. Tonsils, lymph nodes, neck muscles
10. Mastoid process
11. Rest of head
12. Cerebrum
13. Cerebellum
14. Temporal lobe
15. Base of skull
16. Top of head
17. Mastoid process
18. Side of neck and head
19. Jaw/teeth (all toes)
20. Nose
21. Naso-pharynx, throat
22. Drain plug (use after G7)
23. A dessert comes next.

B. Other Toes

1. Sinuses
2. Eustachian tube
3. Side of neck
4. Lymphatics, head and neck
5. Coping reflexes
6. Ears
7. Eyes
8. And now a dessert

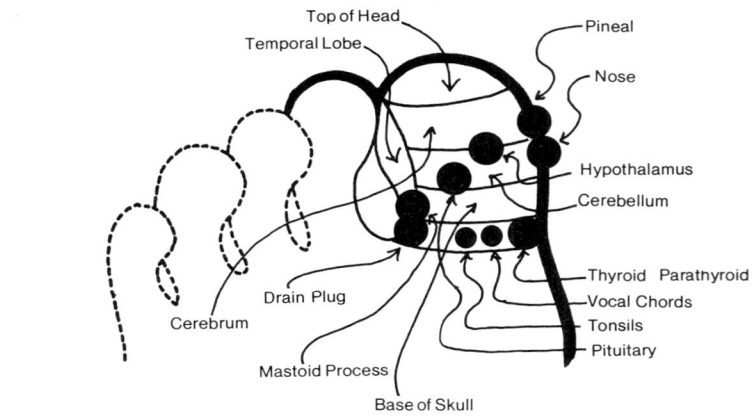

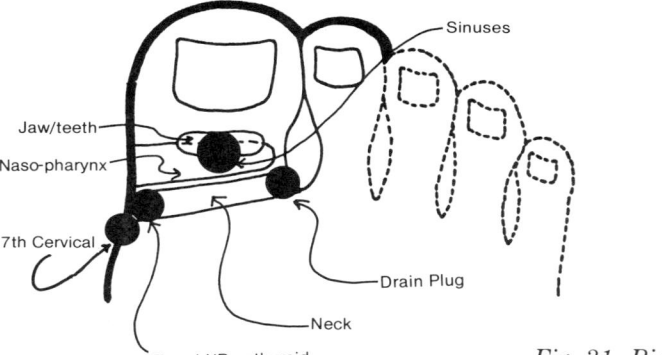

Fig. 31. Big Toe Reflexes

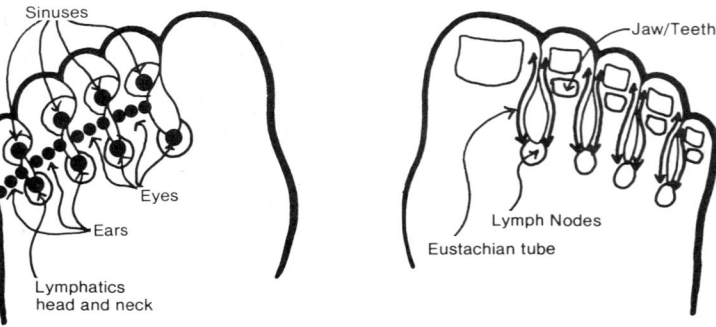

Fig. 32. Other Toe Reflexes

C Ball of the foot

1. Lymphatics, head and neck
2. Eyes and ears
3. Shoulder muscles
4. Skin
5. Lymphatic pull across shoulder reflex
6. Shoulder joint
7. Axillary lymphatics
8. 7th cervical
9. Thoracic spine
10. Sternum
11. Trachea/esophagus
12. Thymus
13. Lung
14. Heart (left foot)
15. Arm
16. Diaphragm
17. Solar plexus
18. A dessert is in order. Now rest your thumb. Go to the dorsum of the foot and use your index and/or other fingers.

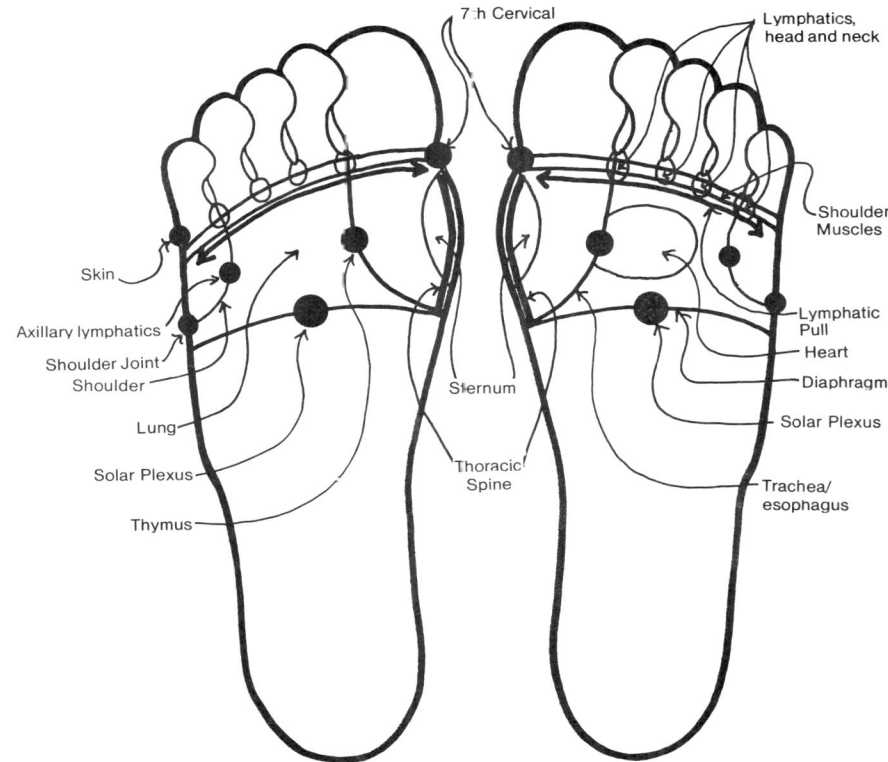

Fig. 33. Ball of the Foot Reflexes

D. Dorsum of the foot

1. Teeth
2. Sinuses
3. Naso-pharynx
4. Back of neck
5. 7th cervical
6. Lymph nodes, head and neck
7. Skin
8. Sternum
9. Bronchials, back muscles, ribs
10. Whiplash, bronchitis reflex
11. Breast
12. Shoulder joint
13. Gall bladder/inner ear
14. Adrenal gland

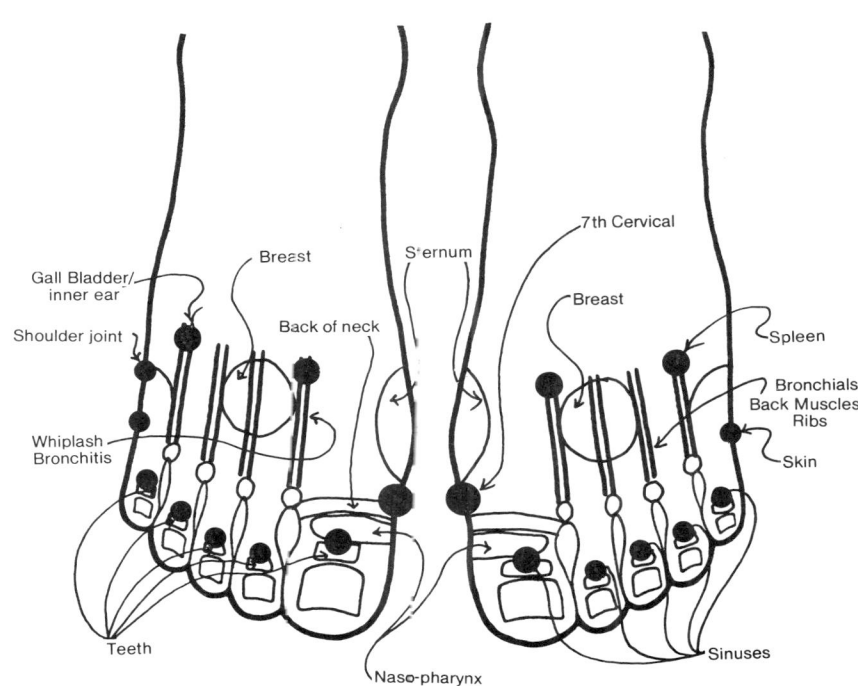

Fig. 34. Dorsum of the Foot Reflexes

E. Arch of foot

1. Arm/thigh/leg
2. Liver (right foot)
3. Gall bladder (right foot)
4. Adrenal
5. Duodenum (right foot)
6. Stomach (mostly left foot)
7. Hiatus Hernia (right foot)
8. Pylorus
9. Pancreas (mostly left foot)
10. Spleen (left foot)
11. Kidney
12. Bladder
13. Ureter tube
14. Ileo-cecal valve and appendix (right foot)
15. Ascending colon (right foot)
16. Transverse colon (right foot)
17. Hepatic flexure (right foot)
18. Splenic flexure (left foot)
19. Small intestine, jujunum, ilium
20. Descending colon (left foot)
21. Sigmoid flexure (left foot)
22. Rectum (left foot)
23. Leg, thigh, arm
24. Follow with stroking and a few desserts.

Note the differences in each foot.

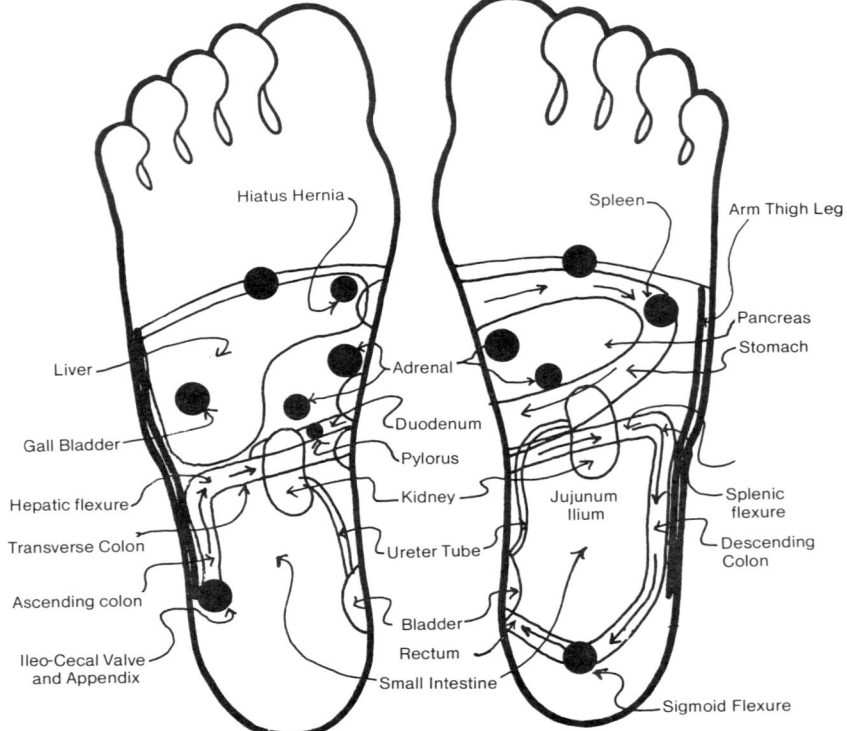

Fig. 35. Arch of the Foot Reflexes

F. Heel of foot

1. Pelvic girdle
2. Sciatic
3. Foot
4. Sigmoid and small intestine (left foot)
5. Hemorrhoid, hip and back pain
6. Lymphatic pull, heel to shoulder joint reflex.

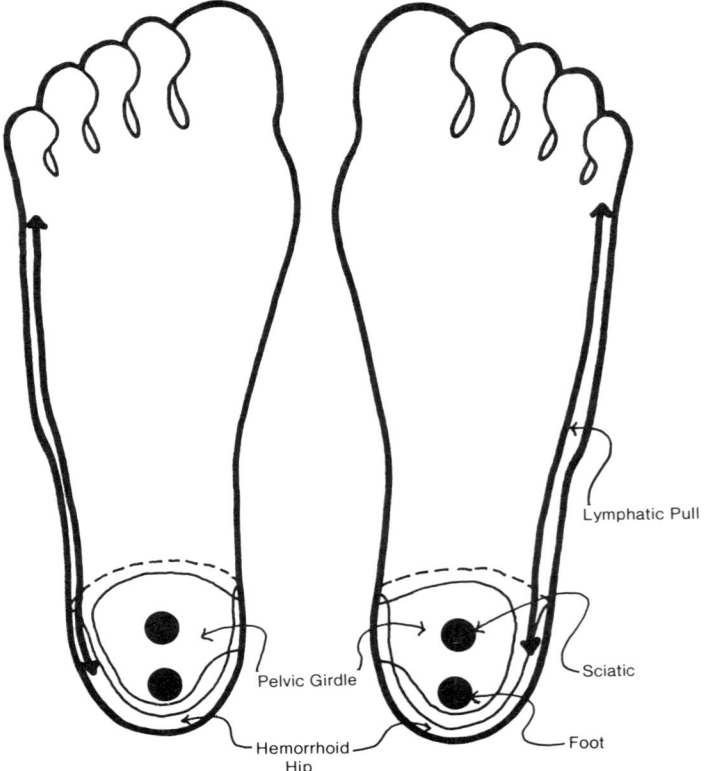

Fig. 36. Heel of the Foot Reflexes

G. Top of foot
Abdominal/groin area, waist to ankle.

1. Inguinal lymph nodes
2. Lymph press/pull
3. Fallopian tube/vas deferens/ inguinal canal
4. Pelvis
5. Symphesis pubis
6. Appendix
7. Lymph drainage (from knee)
8. Drain plug
9. A dessert follows.

H. Medial side of foot
Big toe or arch side

1. Pineal
2. Nose
3. Cervicals
4. 7th Cervical
5. Thoracic
6. Lumbar
7. Sacrum
8. Coccyx
9. Bladder
10. Uterus/prostate
11. Penis/urethra/vagina
12. Rectum
13. Fallopian tube and lymph in groin
14. Hip joint
15. Pelvic girdle and pelvic lymph-atics
16. Rectum (two points)
17. Fallopian tube/vas deferens/ inguinal canal
18. Symphesis pubis
19. Inguinal lymph nodes
20. 7th cervical/coccyx hold

I. Medial side of leg

1. Thigh, knee
2. Menstrual point
3. Spine/colon

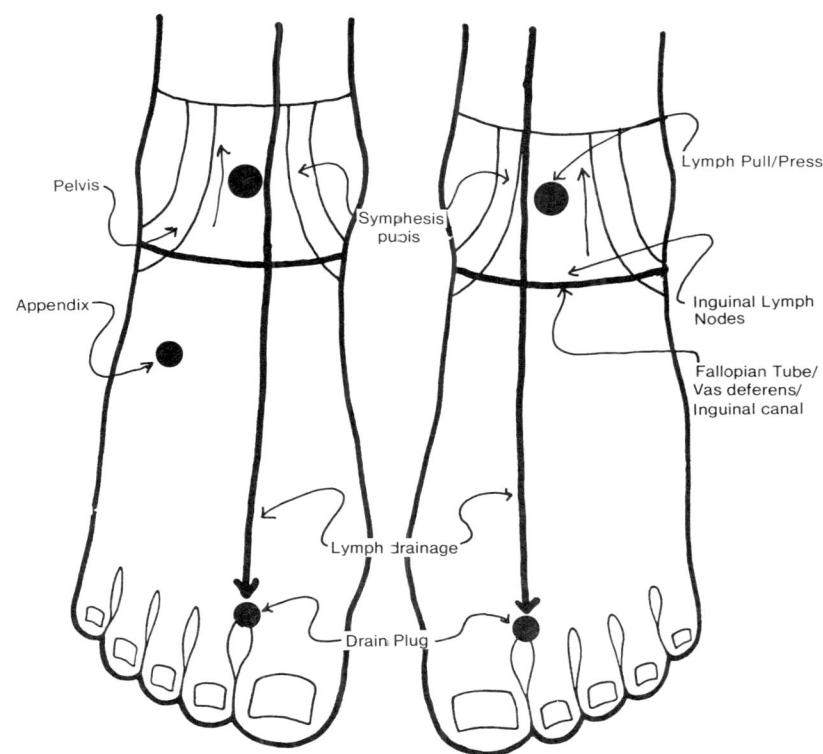

Fig. 37. Top of the Foot Reflexes

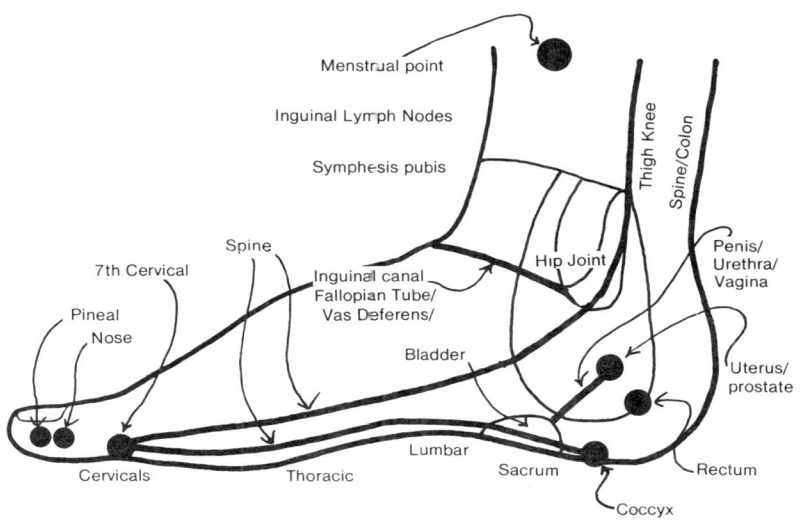

Fig. 38. Medial Side of the Foot Reflexes

147

J. Lateral side of foot (outside)

1. Ear
2. Skin
3. Shoulder joint (2 reflexes)
4. Arm/thigh/leg
5. Waist/elbow/knee
6. Hip/knee/low back
7. Sciatic/hip/low back
8. Pelvic girdle
9. Ovary/testes
10. Buttock
11. Add a dessert before going to:
12. Lateral side of leg, spine, low back
13. Now follow with several desserts.

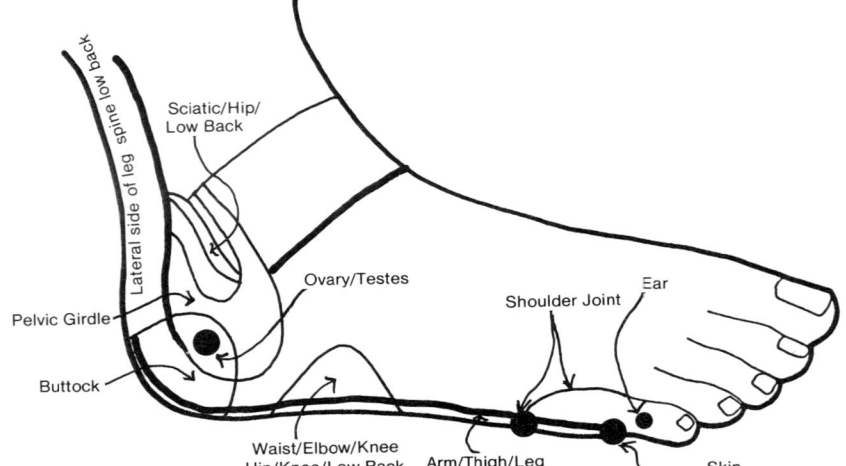

Fig. 39. Lateral Side of the Foot Reflexes

K. End your session with

1. Solar plexus breathing
2. 7th cervical/coccyx
3. Nerve stroke
4. Cleansing stroke

L. Rest — Let your client rest a few moments while you wash up.

M. Help the client — If you have your client seated in a recliner *YOU* tilt it back down. If your client tilts it he may injure his back which you have just relaxed. Anyway, it's a nice thing to do.

N. Back rub — A bit of a back rub serves at least four purposes:
1) it gets your client out of the chair,
2) it feels wonderful, friendly,
3) it relaxes the muscles, energizes the person, and
4) if you know other methodologies (acupuncture, body work, feldenkriess etc...) here's the chance to use them.

O. Work hands — Work the hands now. It reminds the body and the subconscious mind that you mean business! It gives the healing process an extra push in the direction of health.

P. A note to you. — If you are aware of auras (energy field that surrounds you) or believe that there are such things –
When you work with a client or friend pull your aura in. When your aura is out, you are more likely to hold on to another's discomfort, become *drained* or in pain.
How do you do it? Pretend! Hallucinate that you are pulling it in. Try it out. Send your aura out to touch another person. How do you feel? Draw it in, how do you feel? Send it out and ask someone you touched what he or she noticed and ask whether they noticed when you drew it in. Silly? Perhaps – but it works.

Q. Enjoy — Enjoy your session – you will then give joy to yourself and your friend.

R. Remember — Any Reflexology that you do to another you can do to yourself. Remember to work on yourself too!

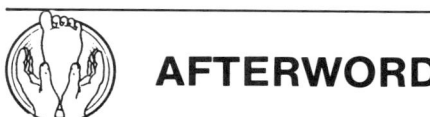

AFTERWORD

I know you've enjoyed this manual – that its information is varied enough to start you on one path while distracting you with another. That is my purpose – BECAUSE THERE IS MORE....

My hope is that your book will become tattered with use as any loved object becomes used and raggedy. May it be for you a "Velveteen Rabbit" loved enough to lose its newness and its shine – but may the subject be ever new, ever bright, and ever delightful.

I would be pleased to hear of your additions, differences, and questions. Address yourself to:

Touchpoint
Canadian Institute of Reflexology & Kinesthetics
49 Queens Street
Port Moody, British Columbia,
V3H 2N3 Canada

Add your name to the mailing list for a newsletter and information on upcoming seminars in Reflexology, Touch For Health Kinesthetics, (Muscle Balancing and Muscle Re-education) and more. Send us your friends' names and we'll send them our newsletter, *Footprints*.

With love we take
OUR FIRST STEP

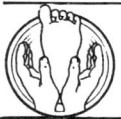

DISCLAIMER

The Touchpoint workbook *The First Steps* and/or the video presentation *The First Steps* are to be used as information only. No item in these pages or in the video presentation is intended as claims for cure and mitigation of disease, or as a diagnostic tool. Your physician has the sole and only right to diagnose and prescribe in health matters. All material herein, of whatever nature or however expressed, is therefore strictly subject to your physician's approval and without recourse or redress in any form to the author or to the publisher.

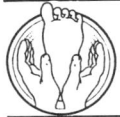

AVAILABLE FROM TOUCHPOINT

Available from Touchpoint, Canadian Institute of Reflexology & Kinesthetics.

Video Home Study Course VHS/BETA "Reflexology - The First Steps"

Look as you listen and learn the reflexes to the entire body. Each reflex is shown in close – both as a point on the foot and how it is worked. Explanations are shown both on a model and an actual foot. See an entire session performed. Functions of all organs and glands explained. Music sets the pace. This video makes it possible for individuals or study groups to learn at your own pace in your own home. Yvette Eastman is your personal instructor. Packaged with or without Manual.

Reflexology Manual "Touchpoint Reflexology The First Steps"

Included in the Video Presentation or on its own this is a state of the art manual, with the most complete and up to date information on Reflexology for both the novice and the experienced practitioner. Hundreds of photographs and illustrations facilitate your learning. Its 28 chapters include old and new reflexes on feet, hand, head and body, use of vitamins, herbs, colour, polarity and even emotions that contribute to dis-ease. A must for your reference library.

Wall Chart 2x3 feet The Foot Chart

Photographic view of all the reflexes, colour coded by system, on superior paper with hanger. Can be obtained laminated or plain.

Wall Chart 2x3 feet The Hand Chart

New from Touchpoint, for those who can't reach their feet or who want to add to the work they do. Old and new reflexes of the hand. Laminated or plain.

Wallet Card of the Reflexes

Foot and hand reflexes in a convenient, easily available fold-over card.

Touchpoint Button

A delightful symbol of your profession – a neat way to recognise another Reflexology person and to attract interest.

Touchpoint T-Shirt

Humorous reflexes let you and your friends laugh their way to better health. Nose reflex is a vacuum cleaner.

Reflexology Wheel

Locate specific reflexes for specific discomforts by turning the wheel.

Learning Tapes (Cassette)

Learn the reflexes while you relax to soothing music and sounds of nature, voiced over with all of the reflexes and relaxation exercises. Learn while you sleep or drive.

Basic Reflexology Certification Seminar

Become a certified Reflexologist. A joyful learning experience. Accelerated learning techniques allow for swift learning and easy retention. Certified Reflexologists receive *Footprints* newsletter and referrals and know that they have achieved a high standard in Reflexology.

Advanced Reflexology Instructional Methods

Advanced techniques, more reflexes, use of additional techniques to aid in better health both for self and others, techniques for enlarging your practise and for teaching reflexology in schools and community centres. Pre-requisite; Basic Reflexology Certification Seminar.

Seminar Muscle Kinesthetics (Touch For Health)

Learn to balance the body's energies, the flow of energy in the muscles, for better posture, pain relief, improved health, emotional stress relief and more using acupressure, Neuro-vascular and neuro-lymphatic points as well as massage techniques.

Mind/Body Seminar

How to heal **your** body by understanding **your** mind. Learn to change your mind, how, why and in what specific direction to reach your highest potential in any endeavour.

Learning Enhancement Workshops (Edu-Kinesthetics)

Learn to learn better even if you believe you have poor recall. Incredible results for slow learners and dyslexics.

Touchpoint *Footprints*

Touchpoint's own newletter, filled with information on new reflexes, new methodologies, nutrition aids to whole body health as well as an up to date referral list of reflexologists and kinesthologists in your area.

Touchpoint
2342 Clarke Road
Port Moody, B.C.
V3H 1Y8
(604) 936-3227

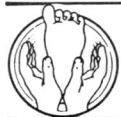

SUGGESTED READING AND BIBLIOGRAPHY

Acupressure - Acupuncture Without Needles, J.V. Cerney
Prentice - Hall, Inc., 1978

Alive Polarity, Jefferson Campbell
Alive Polarity Publications, 1982

The Anatomy Coloring Book, Wynn Kapt/Lawrence M.
Elson, Harper & Row Publishers, Inc., 1977

*Are You Tense? The Benjamin System of Muscular
Therapy,* Ben E. Benjamin
Random House, Inc., 1978

The Art of Seeing, Aldous Huxley
Montana Books, Publishers, Inc.

The Art of Seeing, Aldous Huxley
Harper & Row, Publishers, Inc., 1975

Athletes' Feet, Editors of Runner's World Magazine
World Publications, 1974

Atlas of Human Anatomy, Samual Smith
Harper & Row, Publishers, 1961

Be Your Own Chiropractor, John & Margaret Barton
Copy Quick, 1979

Behold Man, Lennart Nilsson
Little, Brown and Company, Ltd., 1974

Better Eyesight Without Glasses, W.H. Bates
Jove Publications, Inc., 1979

Better Health with Foot Reflexology, Dwight Byers
Ingham Publications Inc., 1983

The Bloodstream, Isaac Asimov
Macmillan Publishing Co., Inc., 1976

The Body Has A Head, Gustav Eckstein
Harper & Row Publishers, Inc., 1970

The Body Has Its Reasons, Therese Bertherat & Carol
Bernstein
Random House, Inc., 1977

Body Reflexology, Mildred Carter
Parker Publishing Company, 1983

The Body Says Yes, Priscilla Kapel
A.C.S. Publications, 1981

The Chemicals of Life, Isaac Asimov
The New American Library, Inc., 1954

The Chinese Art of Healing, Stephan Palos,
Herder & Herder, Inc., 1971

Color Healing, collection,
Health Research, 1956

Color Power, Dorothea L. Mella
Domel Artbooks, 1981

Color Therapy, Dr. Reuben Amber
A.S.I. Publishers Inc., 1980

The Complete Book of Natural Medicines, David Carroll
Summit Books, 1980

The Complete Guide to Foot Reflexology, Kevin & Barbara
Kunz
Prentice - Hall, Inc., 1980

Dreams and Healing, John A. Sanford
Paulist Press, 1978

Dr. Schuessler's Biochemistry, J.B. Chapman
New Era Laboratories Ltd., 1973

Doctor-Patient Handbook, Bernard Jensen
BiWorld Publishers Inc., 1976

The Doctor's Book of Vitamin Therapy, Harold Rosenberg
& A.N. Feldzamen
G.P. Putnam's Sons, 1974

Ear Acupressure, Pedro Chan
Chan's Corporation, 1977

Encyclopedia of Natural Remedies, J. Merril Harmon
Kosman Publishing, Inc., 1978

An Endocrine Interpretation of Chapman's Reflexes, The
Interpreter
American Academy of Osteopathy, 1980

First Aid Using Simple Remedies, Michael Blate
Falkynor Books, 1982

Food is Your Best Medicine, Henry G. Beiler
Random House Inc., 1965

The Foot Book, Advice for Athletes, Harry F. Hlavac
World Publication, Inc., 1977

The Foot Book, Healing the Body Through Reflexology,
Devaki Berkson
Harper & Row Publishers Inc., 1977

Foot Reflexology, Ina Bryant
O'Sullivan, Woodside & Co., 1981

The G-Jo Handbook, Michael Blate
Falkynor Books, 1976

Good Hands - Massage Techniques for Total Health,
Robert Bahr
New American Library, Ltd., 1984

A Guide to Physical Examination, Barbara Bates
J B. Lippincott Company, 1974

Hand Reflexology: Key to Perfect Health, Mildred Carter
Parker Publishing Company, Inc., 1975

The Handbook of Alternatives to Chemical Medicine,
Mildred Jackson & Terri Teague
Terri K. Teague & Mildred Jackson, N.D., 1975

Handbood of Unusual and Unorthodox Healing Methods,
J.V. Cerney
Parker Publishing Company, Inc., 1976

Healing Energies, Stephen Paul Shepard
  Hawthorne Books, 1981

Healing For The Age Of Enlightenment, Stanley Burroughs
  Stanley Burroughs, 1976

Healing Herbs for Arthritis and Rheumatism, Alexandra Donson
  Fforbez Publications, 1982

The Health Finder, J.I. Rodale
  Rodale Books, Inc., 1955

Helping Your Health With Pointed Pressure Therapy, Roy E. Bean
  Parker Publishing Company, Inc., 1975

Helping Yourself With Foot Reflexology, Mildred Carter
  Parker Publishing Company, Inc., 1974

The Herb Book, John Lust
  Benedict Lust Publications, 1974

Holistic H.E.L.P. Handbook, Stanley Steven Kalson
  International Holistic Centre, Inc., 1981

How to Get Well, Paavo Airola
  Health Plus Publishers, 1977

How to Heal Yourself Using Foot Acupressure (Foot Reflexology), Michael Blate
  Falkynor Books, 1982

Human Anatomy & Physiology, David LeVay
  Coles Publishing Company Limited, 1978

The Human Body, Paul Lewis and David Rubenstein
  Bantam Books, 1972

The Human Body - Its Structure and Operation, Isaac Asimov
  The New American Library, Inc., 1963

The Human Brain, Isaac Asimov
  The New American Library, Inc., 1965

Human Physiology, Arthur J. Vander/James H. Sherman/Dorothy S. Luciano
  McGraw-Hill Book Company, 1975

The Johns Hopkins Atlas of Human Functional Anatomy, George D. Zuidema
  The Johns Hopkins University Press, 1978

Listen to Your Pain, Ben D. Benjamin
  Penguin Books, 1984

Medicinal Herbs (Encyclopedia of), Joseph Kadans
  Arco Publishing Company, Inc., 1972

Mental and Elemental Nutrients, Carl C. Pfeiffer
  Keats Publishing, Inc., 1975

Mind as Healer, Mind as Slayer, Kenneth R. Pelletier
  Dell Publishing Co., Inc., 1978

The Miracle of Metaphysical Healing, Evelyn M. Monahan
  Parker Publishing Company, Inc., 1975

Mirror of the Body, Anna Kaye & Don C. Matchan
  Strawberry Hill Press, 1978

Modern Home Medical Adviser, Morris Fishbein
  Doubleday & Company, Inc., 1969

Muscle Response Test, Walter Fischman/Mark Grinims
  Richard Marek Publishers, 1979

The Nature Doctor, A. Vogel
  Bioforce - Verlag Teufen (AR), 1952

Nature Has a Remedy, Bernard Jensen
  Bernard Jensen, D.C., 1978

Natural Healing (The Practical Encyclopedia of), Mark Bricklin
  Rodale Press, Inc., 1976

A New Breed of Doctor, Alan H. Nittler
  Pyramid Publications, 1977

Of Men and Plants, Maurice Messegue
  Macmillan Publishing Co., Inc.

The Oliver Method of New Body Reflexology, William H. Oliver
  Bi - World Publishers, 1976

On Your Feet, Elizabeth H. Roberts
  Rodale Press, 1980

Oriental Diagnosis, Michio Kushi,
  Sunwheel Publication, 1980

Own Your Own Body, Stan Malstrom
  Fresh Mountain Air Publishing Company, 1978

Pain Erasure, Bonnie Prudden
  Ballantine Books, 1982

The Patient, Not the Cure, Margery G. Blackie,
  Woodbridge Press Publishing Company, 1978

Photographic Anatomy of the Human Body, C. Yokochi, J. W. Rohen
  University Park Press, 1978

Psycho Dietetics, E. Cheraskin, W.M. Ringsdorf Jr., Arline Brecher
  Stein and Day Publishers, 1974

The Rainbow In Your Hands, Albert Roy Davis, Walter C. Rawls, Jr.
  Exposition Press, Inc., 1977

Reflexology, Maybelle Segal
  Wilshire Book Company, 1978

Reflexology Today, Doreen E. Bayly
  Thorsons Publishers Limited, 1982

Reflex Zone Therapy of the Feet, Hanne Marquardt
  Thorsons Publishers, Inc., 1983

Relief from Pain with Finger Massage, Roger Dalet
  Hutchinson & Co. Ltd., 1979

Schick Notebook Charts
  Caroline House Publishers

The Science of Practice of Iridology, Bernard Jensen
  Bernard Jensen, 1974

Simple Relaxation, Laura Mitchell
John Murray Publishers Ltd., 1977

Stories the Feet Can Tell Through Reflexology, Eunice D.
Ingham
Ingham Publishings Inc., 1938

Stories the Feet Have Told Through Refleoxology, Eunice
D. Ingham
Ingham Publishings Inc., 1963

Switching On, Paul E. Dennison
Edu-Kinesthetics, Inc., 1981

The Therapeutic Touch, Dolores Krieger
Prentice Hall, Inc., 1979

Tissue Cleansing through Bowel Management, Bernard
Jensen
Bernard Jensen, 1981

Touch for Health, John F. Thie,
DeVorss & Co. Publishers, 1979

Way to Natural Health and Beauty, Maurice Messegue
MacMillan Publishing Co., Inc., 1974

Wholistic Healing, Elan Z. Neev
Ageless Books, 1977

Wireless Anatomy of Man and Its Functions, Randolph
Stone
CRCS Publications, 1978

You Can Master Disease, Bernard Jensen
Bernard Jensen, Publishing Division, 1976

You Don't Have to Ache: Orthotherapy, Arthur A. Michele
M. Evans and Company, Inc., 1971

Your Body and How It Works, J.D. Ratcliff
Reader's Digest Press/Delacorte Press, 1976

Your Healing Hands, Richard Gordon
Unity Press, 1978

Zone Reflex, Joe Shelby Riley
Health Research, 1961

Zone Therapy, Wm. H. Fitzgerald/Edwin F. Bowers/
George Starr White
Health Research, 1978

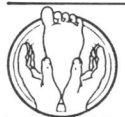

INDEX

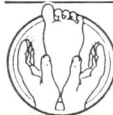

COPY FOR YOUR FILES

Mark the sensitive areas that you find on the person and keep a copy in your files so that you may have a record of the person's progress.

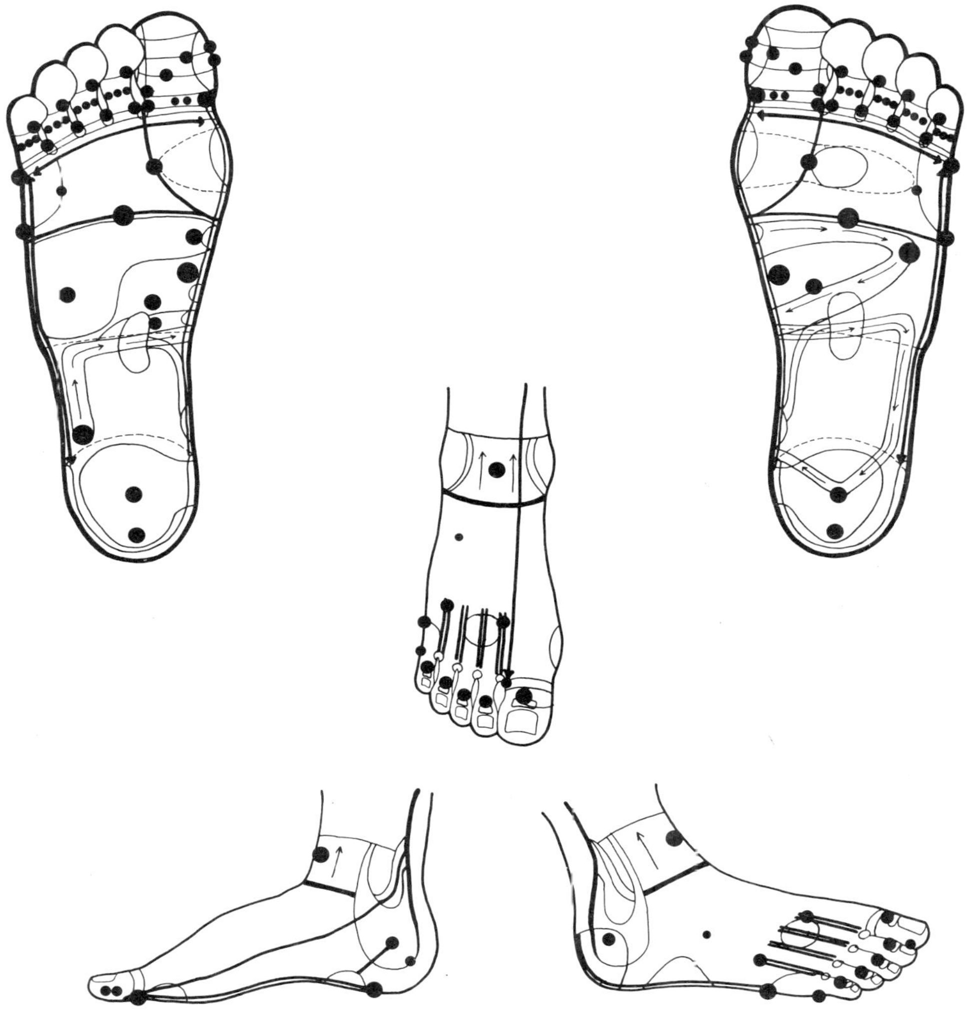

Date _____

Medications_____

_____

Supplements _____

Name _____

Address _____

Phone _____ Phone _____

Comments _____

_____